THE
DIABETES
BREAK-
THROUGH

THE
DIABETES
BREAK-
THROUGH

BASED ON A SCIENTIFICALLY PROVEN PLAN TO REVERSE DIABETES THROUGH WEIGHT LOSS

Osama Hamdy, M.D., Ph.D.,
and Sheri R. Colberg, Ph.D.

WM

WILLIAM MORROW

An Imprint of HarperCollins*Publishers*

HarperCollins books may be purchased for educational, business, or sales promotional use. For information please e-mail the Special Markets Department at SPsales@harpercollins.com.

A hardcover edition of this book was published in 2013 by Harlequin Enterprises, Ltd.

FIRST WILLIAM MORROW PAPERBACK EDITION PUBLISHED 2015.

The Library of Congress has cataloged the hardcover edition as follows:

Library of Congress Cataloging-in-Publication Data
Hamdy, Osama.
   The diabetes breakthrough : a scientifically proven program to lose weight, cut medications and reverse diabetes / Osama Hamdy M.D., Ph.D., and Sheri R. Colberg, Ph.D.
      pages cm
   Includes index.
   Summary: "A senior Harvard Medical School diabetologist and top exercise physiologist share a proven and effective 12-week plan to reverse diabetes, lose weight and ditch the medi-cation for good." -- Provided by publisher.
   ISBN 978-0-373-89284-6 (hardback)
   1. Diabetes—Alternative treatment. 2. Diabetics—Rehabilitation. 3. Weight loss. I. Colberg, Sheri, 1963- II. Title.
   RC661.A47H34 2013
   616.4'620654—dc23

                  2013040236

ISBN 978-0-06-240719-1 (pbk.)

15 16 17 18 19 [OV/RRD] 10 9 8 7 6 5 4 3 2 1

In memory of my parents, who died from diabetes before I knew how to help them

–Osama Hamdy

In loving memory of my maternal grandmother, Velda Huffman Stubbs, for whom this program was not developed soon enough

–Sheri Colberg

CONTENTS

PART I — THE DIABETES SOLUTION

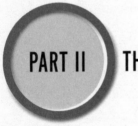

PART II THE DIABETES LIFE PLAN

Foreword by John L. Brooks III
President and Chief Executive Officer,
Joslin Diabetes Center

I am deeply honored to write this foreword for *The Diabetes Breakthrough*, as this book provides a practical and essential home-based approach to enabling those with or at risk of diabetes to achieve lasting weight loss and a lifetime of living well. It is interesting to note the recent declaration by the American Medical Association that obesity is a disease. This recognition further highlights the urgent need for addressing this disease, as we clearly understand how obesity and one's lifestyle cause diabetes and all of its devastating and costly complications. The United States Centers for Disease Control and Prevention estimates that over one-third of Americans are obese. The World Health Organization estimates that 35 percent of adults worldwide are overweight and 11 percent are obese. Clearly, we have a true global pandemic, but through the remarkable insights of Drs. Hamdy and Colberg, and the demonstrated success of the Why WAIT program, *The Diabetes Breakthrough* shows patients and consumers from all walks of life how to approach weight loss and lifestyle modifications in a step-by-step, personalized fashion.

Rich with proven motivational techniques and easy to understand and assimilate steps, *The Diabetes Breakthrough*'s 12-week Diabetes Solution assuredly gets everyone on a solid path for continuing and sustainable success. Then its Diabetes Life Plan will ensure that the habits and positive results delivered over the participant's past three months are maintained for a lifetime.

I am confident that this book will make a real and impactful difference, as it was born out of the personal passions and convictions of its two devoted and gifted authors to change the course of events for those living with diabetes, and those at risk of developing diabetes. This book will truly change lives— for the better!

ACKNOWLEDGMENTS

The Why WAIT program would not be possible without the enormous help and creativity of many of my colleagues at the Joslin Diabetes Center, Harvard Medical School and throughout the greater diabetes research community. I would like to thank John L. Brooks III, the Joslin president and CEO, whose vision of a world free of diabetes and its complications supports the Why WAIT program. He is tirelessly leading Joslin efforts to achieve its mission to prevent, treat and cure diabetes.

I am deeply indebted to Dr. Ron Kahn, the pioneer researcher, Joslin chief academic officer and past CEO of the Joslin Diabetes Center, who encouraged me to start the Joslin Clinical Obesity Program and to think outside the box for better nutritional tools that can effectively impact diabetes control. I also want to thank several great former and current leaders at Joslin clinic, including Dr. Alan Moses, the former chief medical officer, Dr. Martin Abrahamson, senior vice president and former chief medical officer, Cathy Carver, vice president for Advocacy and Planning, Dr. Robert Gabbay, chief medical officer, and Bridget Stewart, vice president for Clinic Operations. Without their unrivaled effort, this program would have remained just an idea. They continued to help in expanding the outreach of the Why WAIT program to benefit every diabetes patient across the globe. I am also grateful to Dr. Edward Horton, the senior investigator at Joslin and past president of the American Diabetes Association, who guided all my clinical research, which led to the strong scientific evidence behind the Why WAIT program.

My heartfelt appreciation goes to the Why WAIT team, a real family of experts who have successfully carried this mission over many years. They never spare any effort in helping our patients get the maximum benefit of this important model for diabetes care. Their innovative approaches have kept this program first class and made it incomparable to any other medically supervised weight management program. From this terrific team, past and present, I want to acknowledge the efforts of Gillian Arathuzik, Dr. Ann Goebel Fabbri, Jaqueline Shahar, Jo-Anne Rizzotto, Dr. Nuha El Sayed, Joan Beaton, Amanda Kirpitch, John Zrebiec, Elisha Phelan, Laura Schwab, Jeffrey Richard, Dr. Amr Morsi and Dr. Adham Mottalib.

There are many others at Joslin and Harvard Medical School who deserve mention for their incredible work, but the list is simply too long to include here.

Above all, I would like to thank all the past and current participants of the Why WAIT program who have inspired us with their successes in battling and overcoming diabetes through effective and long-lasting weight loss. To them and to every individual with diabetes, I would like to introduce this book.—O.H.

On behalf of Dr. Hamdy and myself, I would like to express many thanks to our literary agent, Linda Konner, and the savvy editor of Harvard Health Publications, Dr. Julie Silver, who has been 100 percent behind this book since its conception. Moreover, we are fully indebted to all the members of the hardworking crew at Harlequin Nonfiction, including our editor, Deborah Brody, who helped us bring this book to all the people with diabetes who can benefit from it.—S.C.

Who would ever have imagined that the often relentless progression of a chronic disease like type 2 diabetes can be stopped or reversed? Or that you can reduce your diabetes medications even if you've been taking multiple ones for a long time, including insulin? The good news for you—and the rapidly expanding number of people with type 2 diabetes worldwide—is that it is finally imaginable and definitely possible and the program outlined in this book is the key to making it happen.

Maybe your doctor just told you that you have a "touch" of the sugar. Is that a reason to worry that you have diabetes? If truth be told, even if you only have a condition called *prediabetes* (which develops before type 2 diabetes), now is the time to get motivated and take action to improve your health and prevent it from turning into full-blown diabetes. Even in the early stages, diabetes can be a treacherous disease, one that may be damaging your blood vessels, eyes and nerves when you don't know you have it and while you're still feeling just fine. Once it has finally been diagnosed, your health may already be starting to suffer.

So what can you do? Luckily, type 2 diabetes is a controllable condition if you lose weight and follow a healthy lifestyle plan. You may have already heard that advice from your doctor, but you may not know how to accomplish these goals. Healthy lifestyle changes, like changing what you eat and exercising more, are critical for controlling diabetes at any stage of the disease, and they're particularly important in the early stages. Improving your lifestyle is also the key to losing enough weight to reverse the course of diabetes and avoid its negative impact on your health and well-being. All you need is the right guide on your path toward conquering it for good. The scientifically proven program you'll find in this book is especially designed to help you do just that.

A HOME-BASED VERSION OF THE "WHY WAIT" PROGRAM FOR YOU

Dr. Hamdy and his team designed a medically managed weight loss program for people with diabetes called "Why **WAIT**" (**W**eight **A**chievement and **I**ntensive **T**reatment), which is offered on-site through the Joslin Diabetes Center in Boston, which is affiliated with Harvard Medical School. This program has resulted in unsurpassed success for its participants—in fact, it's the only clinical program to show long-term successful weight loss for people with diabetes. In 2015, the American Diabetes Association gave Dr. Hamdy and his Why WAIT team the prestigious Michaela Modan Award for conducting the best human study in the epidemiology, prevention and management of diabetes. This study showed the 5-year results of the Why WAIT program, where participants maintained significant weight loss. In the same year, the *Journal of Clinical Endocrinology and Metabolism* published a study that showed comparable results between the Why WAIT program and bariatric surgery after one year of intervention. Even though you'll be doing this home-based version of the Joslin Why WAIT program called the *Diabetes Breakthrough* on your own, it will help you lose and keep the weight off if you follow the program as closely as you possibly can.

We've known for a while that improving your lifestyle to help you lose as little as 10 or 15 pounds can prevent type 2 diabetes in the first place. But Dr. Hamdy and his colleagues at the Joslin Diabetes Center showed that losing a similar amount of weight (around 7 percent of your total body weight) can rev up your insulin action and frequently reverse the course of type 2 diabetes or prevent the development of health problems associated with it. Participants who went through the 12-week Why WAIT program at Joslin were able to cut their medications by an average of 50 to 60 percent and many of them were able to go off medications entirely, all while keeping their diabetes in great control.

It's time you joined them on the path to better health, a lesser chance of drug side effects and more money in your pocket as a result of paying for fewer expensive medications. Even if you don't reach your goal weight or completely eliminate your medications, how would you like to live a longer and healthier life without carrying around all those extra pounds? Our results at Joslin show it's possible and in this book you will learn how to make it happen for you.

What makes this program so unique? Here are ten innovations that make it a true breakthrough for weight loss and health management for anyone with diabetes or prediabetes:

1. This program progresses over 12 weeks like no other, with doable increases in your exercise plan, effective ways to change your bad habits and transitions in your diet from replacing some of your meals with meal shakes to eating just regular foods.

2. It's not just about reducing your calories by a set amount or eating only a certain amount of fat to lose weight; instead, you will be assigned a specific calorie level regardless of your current daily calories and you will follow a unique dietary plan that includes eating more protein and the choice of carbohydrates that cause smaller glucose spikes.

3. You'll learn how to combine eating healthy foods and meal replacement shakes, both with specific proportions of carbohydrates, protein and fat to better manage your blood glucose levels and body weight.

4. On this program, you'll be able to eat many of your regular foods following our special menus that were developed from commonly used foods (instead of making you eat new foods you may not like or follow strange and unusual menus).

5. Your activity plan has a greater emphasis on strength exercise to build muscle, not just cardio workouts like most weight loss plans.

6. Unlike most plans, you'll work up to doing about 300 minutes of weekly exercise that fits into your daily lifestyle (in comparison to more common recommendations of only 150 minutes of weekly cardio exercise).

7. Through this book, your health care providers will have access to algorithms that offer guidelines for precisely changing your diabetes medications to enhance weight loss, especially to avoid hypoglycemia (low blood glucose levels).

8. You'll also learn why you should consult with your health care team about revisiting the dosages and types of diabetes medications you take as you lose weight and you'll find out why it's important to continue to monitor your blood glucose levels.

9. You'll learn a lot about how to change your habits and the behaviors that caused you to gain weight in the first place.

10. In addition to learning about how to lose weight safely, this program also teaches you everything you need to know about managing your diabetes more effectively.

COULD THIS BE YOUR STORY?

We'd like you to meet Linda, a graduate of the revolutionary Joslin Why WAIT program. Her story is that she started out at a normal weight when she was a young adult, but over the next four decades she steadily added about a pound a year, gaining over 40 pounds total and developing type 2 diabetes in the process. She had a family history of diabetes, but it was her weight gain and lifestyle that contributed to her development of type 2 diabetes.

Naturally, she tried to lose the weight after she got the bad news, especially since her doctor kept emphasizing the need to lower her weight to control her blood glucose levels. Linda knew how to lose weight on a diet; in fact, she repeatedly dieted and exercised over a decade when her weight gain had become embarrassing to her, but without any lasting success. She was worried that this time wouldn't be any different. Basically, despite what she had heard about the program, she expected to drop some pounds and then eventually gain it back again like she always had in the past—only now she also had diabetes to contend with and that wasn't going away.

WHAT ARE YOU THINKING?

How does Linda's story relate to your own? Have you been gaining weight slowly over the years? How many times have you lost weight on a diet, only to gain it all back—and maybe some extra—not long after? Do you dread the holidays every year since you know you'll pack on more weight? How much weight had you gained by the time you found out that you now have type 2 diabetes to deal with, as well?

Let's find out what you're thinking. How many of the following statements describe something you've said or thought at one time or another?

- "I weigh more than I want to."
- "I know I need to lose some weight."
- "My doctor told me I have to lose some weight."
- "I'm on a diet (or I was recently)."
- "I felt better both physically and mentally after I lost weight."
- "I weigh more now than when I started my first diet."
- "I'm totally discouraged about keeping the weight off and I think it's impossible."
- "I really don't know what I should be eating anymore."
- "I don't know which diet to try next."
- "I'm depressed about how much I weigh."
- "I hate the way my body looks."
- "I think about food and eating all the time."
- "I don't get enough exercise."
- "I know I need to be more active."
- "My doctor told me I need to exercise more."
- "I already broke my New Year's resolution to exercise more."
- "I may have to have surgery to lose weight."
- "My doctor keeps increasing my diabetes pills."
- "I'm taking more insulin than ever before, but my blood glucose is still high."

If even one of these comments applies to you, then this Diabetes Breakthrough program is your tool to achieve what you've been dreaming of for yourself.

THE REAL PROBLEM WITH DIETS

You may already know from experience that losing weight on a diet may not be enjoyable, but it is usually possible. With everyone dieting, why are people around the world generally getting heavier instead of thinner? The real dieting dilemma is that fad diets have no scientific basis. New diet books come out all the time and you can walk into any bookstore and find dozens of different ones to choose from. If you search an online bookseller, you'll find hundreds of options. This abundance of unproven dieting methods makes an incredibly important topic extremely confusing for everyone trying to sort out fact from fiction related to dieting.

A major problem with many of these fad diets that promote rapid weight loss by severely cutting calories is that they can lead to a medically dangerous condition called starvation ketosis, which occurs when your body ineffectively attempts to burn fat when your carbohydrate or calorie intake is very low and is specifically harmful for people with diabetes. What's more, most very low-fat diets lead you to eat less protein than you need and cause you to lose too much muscle mass in the process.

Another major issue with fad diets is that they are usually too extreme—for example, many eliminate entire food groups like grains and other carbohydrates—for people to actually be able to continue on them for long. A study done at Tufts Medical Center comparing these diets found that at the end of a year, dieters' average weight loss is not more than three pounds since most people can't stay on these diets for more than a few weeks.

A common underlying philosophy of these diets is that if you take in fewer calories than you burn off, you'll lose weight. However, healthy weight loss is not that simple. If you diet by reducing calories using an unhealthy nutrition plan (such as the latest fad diet), you'll lose weight—and then you'll almost assuredly gain it back. Now not only are you heavier than ever, but you're also likely "fatter" than before you went on your first diet, meaning that your percent body fat (the relative amount of fat compared to your total weight) is probably higher than ever. Why? It results from losing weight too rapidly using the wrong dietary balance without exercising and subsequently gaining the weight back, which 90 to 95 percent of dieters eventually do.

Following these fad diets, you're likely to lose 10 pounds or even more in the first week or two; however, most of it is water weight, which is why it's also so easy to gain that back when you start eating more normally again. If you continue losing weight at the recommended rate of one to two pounds per week after the first week or so, you'll likely be losing both fat and muscle. On the contrary, if you are eating enough protein and exercising regularly while dieting, you will shift the weight loss to losing mostly fat (which you want to lose) instead of muscle (which you definitely want to keep).

KEEP THE MUSCLE—OR ELSE

Why is keeping your muscle when you lose weight so important? Although the weight lost on most diets is a combination of both fat and muscle, what you gain back afterward is usually just fat (with little or no muscle regain). Going through that cycle repeatedly can contribute to a poorer quality of life and a worsening of your blood glucose control due to loss of muscle. Everyone tends to lose some muscle mass just from getting older as well, so losing it for both reasons is a double whammy to your metabolism and glucose control since muscle is where you burn calories and store most of the extra carbohydrates that you eat.

Aging combined with diabetes is an even worse scenario. Most people who don't have diabetes lose about half a pound of muscle a year as they age. However, if you have diabetes, you lose closer to three-quarters or a full pound of muscle with each passing year. If your diabetes is undiagnosed or poorly controlled, you may be losing more than a pound a year. Eventually, your muscles will get weaker, which will limit your activity and reduce the quality of daily living. When you go on a typical weight loss diet, you will lose about three pounds of muscle for every ten pounds you drop. You definitely don't want to lose that much muscle because it's very difficult to get it back. For the best health outcomes, the muscle mass you lose should not exceed 10 to 15 percent of your total weight loss—or no more than one to one and a half pounds out of every 10—especially when you have diabetes, which is only possible if you exercise while losing weight.

The number one rule for being successful at losing weight *and* keeping it off and reversing or improving your diabetes course is that you absolutely have to lose the fat, but keep the muscle—which the dietary composition and the exercise component of this Diabetes Breakthrough program are designed to help you do. For example, by 2013, over 500 Why WAIT program participants with diabetes lost an average of 24 pounds after only 12 weeks, while preserving muscle mass—not many other diets can do that. Our program incorporates the Joslin Nutrition Guidelines, which were initially developed in 2005 with just the right balance of carbohydrate, protein and fat to achieve proven benefits for body weight and diabetes control. If you attempt to lose body fat by simultaneously eating the right combination of foods, changing your behaviors, exercising regularly and modifying your medications, you'll be a lot less likely to regain the weight you lose.

The Diabetes Breakthrough Is Not a Diet—It's a Lifestyle

This program is not a diet in the traditional sense (although it does cut calories), but is more appropriately considered guidance to revamp your lifestyle so that you lose weight and keep it off. Compare the differences:

TYPICAL WEIGHT LOSS DIET	DIABETES BREAKTHROUGH
• Quick, temporary changes	• Long-term, sustainable changes
• Good foods/bad foods	• Moderation is key
• On it or off it	• Flexible food choices
• Sense of deprivation, anger and rebellion	• Constantly working at it
• Short exercise spurts	• Changed attitudes, habits about eating and exercise
	• More active throughout the day

LONG-TERM WEIGHT LOSS SUCCESS AT LAST

Let's get back to Linda's story. At age 62, she was finally able to lose 23 pounds after just 12 weeks in the Joslin Diabetes Center's life-changing Why WAIT program, where she learned how to keep the weight off for good. And keep it off she has—for more than four years already, which is much longer than she ever managed to do after any of the many other diets she tried in the past decade.

How does she do it? "It's all about eating the right food combinations and smaller portions. Now I eat less, but more often—six times a day—which keeps my blood glucose from going too wildly high or low and I rarely feel hungry," Linda declares. "On other diets, I would eat an apple for a snack, thinking I was making a healthy choice. Well, it is—if you don't have diabetes. The program taught me that it's all about getting the right balance of foods, even in snacks. They encouraged me to eat a handful of nuts or another food with protein in it along with my apple to keep my blood glucose more stable." And following this program has worked like a charm for her.

YOU'LL HAVE A BREAKTHROUGH IN MORE WAYS THAN ONE

"What was wrong with all of the other diets I tried is not that I couldn't lose weight," Linda reminisces. "I could. In fact, all the other diets I tried actually worked and I lost some weight. The issue was that none of them ever controlled my blood glucose levels very well." That's just one thing that makes this program so different from the current pack of diets. The Why WAIT program has a proven, phenomenal success rate of 82 percent of participants reaching all their blood glucose goals in just 12 weeks, along with improvements in blood pressure, cholesterol levels, liver and kidney function and more.

What else makes the Why WAIT program a true diabetes breakthrough? Unlike all the "quick fix" programs out there, years of scientific research have gone into developing this program at the Joslin Diabetes Center, the world's premier diabetes treatment facility. Dr. Osama Hamdy, the medical director of the Why WAIT program, has worked with his team of endocrinologists, nurses, dietitians, exercise physiologists and psychologists to perfect a revolutionary approach that leads to lasting weight reduction in people with type 2 diabetes. The program has been tested for over eight years on hundreds of program participants with consistently remarkable results. For example, over 50 percent of former participants have been able to maintain a weight loss of about 10 percent—close to 25 pounds, on average—after four years on their own and have great diabetes control during that time to boot.

What's more, Dr. Hamdy and his colleagues were the first to show that losing about 7 percent of your body weight—the equivalent of only 14 pounds if you start the plan weighing 200 pounds or just over 20 pounds if you're 300 pounds at the beginning—results in a 57 percent improvement in insulin action in people with type 2 diabetes. That means that your insulin is working a whole lot better and you can get by with much less of it (whether you make all of your own or take doses of it).

Each of the 12 weeks of the Diabetes Breakthrough program focuses on key weight loss strategies, smarter medication use, easy-to-follow dietary guidelines, doable exercise and physical activities and behavioral and motivational topics that will help you change your health and your quality of life for the better. You'll master each step of the program, one week at a time. You'll figure out which diabetes medications make you gain weight and how to adjust them (with your doctor's help) to make the pounds fall off. You'll eat a healthy diet, feel better, look better and may be able to stop or reduce most of your medications after the 12 weeks. Finally, you'll start feeling more like yourself again due to the energy you'll have after following the exercise plan and the program in general.

AND YOU CAN EVEN EAT (DARK) CHOCOLATE

Linda is ecstatic about her new, slimmer figure and enthusiastic about how much energy she has now—enough to exercise every day. For her the best part, though, is how these combined changes have made her blood glucose levels perfectly normal again and she's currently free of all her diabetes medications. Most of those other diets she followed were restrictive and time-consuming: count this, add up these points, measure that, avoid this other thing. And none of them let her eat any sweets, not even chocolate.

"What's best about the Why WAIT dietary plan is that nothing is completely taboo, not even chocolate. But it still manages my blood glucose levels so well that it's like my diabetes is gone," Linda says. "I eat dark chocolate daily now, but it's all about portion control, so I just eat one square of it. I get to eat ice cream, too, since all fats aren't considered bad on this program like they are on so many other diets. I eat the little 60-calorie miniature Dove ice cream bars for snacks and I even get to eat two a day... and my blood glucose numbers are still fine. My doctor said I don't even have pre-diabetes anymore, let alone diabetes." Linda is just one of our many similar success stories.

AND IF YOU STILL NEED MORE REASONS TO START NOW

Here are just a few more reasons why this program is the right one for you:

1. You will not feel hungry when following the unique Why WAIT dietary plan.
2. You get to eat delicious and nutritious food selected from the food that you normally eat, but in a structured plan.
3. You may save a lot of money on your medications (past participants in the Why WAIT program saved more than $500 a year on average).

4. You get to drink tasty, ready-made shakes for breakfast and lunch, which is a real timesaver on hectic days.
5. You'll actually fit into some of your old clothes again.
6. You'll finally know how to eat wisely at buffets, restaurants and other people's houses (and avoid overeating for good).
7. You'll have excellent reasons to put your daily exercise at the top of your calendar.
8. Your fiber will come from delicious foods instead of a container.
9. Your superset training will give your muscles definition and you'll look more toned.
10. You can still eat carbohydrates—even pasta and potatoes.

Now that we've told you what the Diabetes Breakthrough program is capable of doing for you, we will guide you step-by-step to help you successfully put into practice this home-based version of the Why WAIT program for yourself. It's likely that by the end of this program, your blood glucose will be better than ever and you will end up using fewer or no medications to control it. All you have to do is keep reading and start following the program precisely as described to reap the benefits.

PART I

THE
DIABETES
SOLUTION

DIABETES BREAKTHROUGH OVERVIEW

Basics about Insulin, Blood Glucose, Calories, Exercise,
Goal-Setting and More

As you may know, type 2 diabetes is partly genetic because your genes make you predisposed to the disease. But lifestyle factors, such as being sedentary, greatly influence whether you get diabetes. Being more physically active can help people with diabetes gain better control of their condition. What's more, healthy lifestyles can prevent type 2 diabetes and reverse prediabetes, as demonstrated by the National Diabetes Prevention Program.

Before you get started on the lifestyle changes that make the Diabetes Breakthrough program so effective, you need a better understanding of how insulin works in your body, how its action relates to diabetes and why this program can slow the progress of diabetes or reverse its course. Once you understand that, following the full 12-week program that follows this chapter will make more sense. We'll also give you an overview of the program so that you'll know what to expect once you get started on it.

WHY DOES INSULIN MATTER SO MUCH?

You may have already heard a lot about insulin, but don't really understand why it is so important in your body. Insulin is a hormone made by the pancreas that, when released into the bloodstream, works like a key that opens the door for the glucose to enter into your cells that are insulin sensitive: primarily muscle, fat and liver cells. During resting conditions, insulin works to make sure that glucose leaves the blood and goes into the cells, the result being that blood glucose drops into a normal range and doesn't go too high or stay elevated for long after you eat.

Glucose for the cells is like the gasoline for your car: both make them run well. If the glucose cannot enter into your cells, however, it will remain trapped in the blood like gasoline in a car's tank that isn't connected to the motor. Unlike gas stuck in a car tank, though, elevated blood glucose unable to enter cells not only makes them work less efficiently, but also causes damage to your body over time.

Two separate, but related, aspects of diabetes are associated with your body's insulin. One aspect is how well the insulin works and the other is how much insulin your body actually produces. In type 2 diabetes, the insulin isn't very effective at getting glucose into the cells, resulting in the insulin resistance state that is very characteristic of that type. Similarly, people with type 1 diabetes can also develop insulin resistance as the result of poor lifestyle habits and weight gain, resulting in a need for higher insulin doses (although in their case, insulin is injected or pumped).

The other aspect is how much insulin the pancreas actually produces. All people with type 1 diabetes are lacking in insulin since their own immune system was triggered to kill their insulin-making pancreatic cells. They must take replacement insulin. However, people with type 2 diabetes may also not make enough insulin, in which case they may need to take oral medications to stimulate the pancreas to produce more or inject some insulin to supplement their body's supply.

In either case, exercise can help your body use insulin more effectively. Moreover, our clinical research at Joslin Diabetes Center has shown that when overweight people with type 2 diabetes lose just 7 percent of their body weight, their insulin sensitivity increases by a stunning 57 percent. This improvement in insulin action means the body needs less insulin to uptake glucose from the blood, which in turn improves diabetes control and reduces the need for medications or even reverses the course of type 2 diabetes, particularly when the duration of this type of diabetes is relatively short.

Which Type of Diabetes Do You Have?

The main types of diabetes are type 1 and type 2. About 10 percent of people who have diabetes have *type 1 diabetes*, a condition in which the pancreas does not make any insulin at all, which is more commonly diagnosed during childhood. The other 90 percent have *type 2 diabetes*, which usually occurs in people who are over 30 years old; however, an increasing number of younger people are struggling with their weight and developing it. Currently around 4 percent of obese adolescents have type 2 diabetes and close to 20 percent of them have prediabetes.

People with type 2 are often (but not always) overweight with a sedentary lifestyle. Other risk factors are high blood pressure, elevated cholesterol and a positive family history. In type 2 diabetes, the body doesn't use insulin well and the pancreas has to produce very large amounts of insulin in order to help the cells use glucose as fuel. However, people with type 1 diabetes are not the only ones who ever use insulin. It is a commonly prescribed medication for many with type 2 diabetes as well and can be an important tool to keep you healthy when prescribed at the right time and in the correct dose.

WHY INSULIN RESISTANCE IS LIKE A BLOCKED KEYHOLE

What is the easiest way to understand the effect of insulin resistance? In your body, think of glucose in the blood as trying to get through the door into the cells. It takes a "key" to open the door, which is insulin and the "keyholes" are the insulin receptors. If the keys and the keyholes are functioning well together, the doors will open and glucose will enter the cells and give them energy to use or store. However, if you don't have enough keys (as in type 1 diabetes) or the keyholes are blocked (type 2), glucose will never pass through the doors and enter the cells, thus remaining high in the blood while the cells are starving. Even if you have more keys (representing more insulin production), when the keyholes are blocked, those keys cannot open any doors. As a consequence, most of the glucose remains in the bloodstream and blood glucose remains high. In the picture that follows illustrating what insulin resistance is like for the cells, the left side of the door represents the bloodstream, while the right side represents the inside of the cells.

How insulin works at rest for someone with type 2 diabetes

In short, type 2 diabetes usually begins when insulin doesn't work well due to insulin resistance. The pancreas will initially try to overcome the resistance by producing more insulin, resulting in a situation called *hyperinsulinemia*. However, insulin is also a growth hormone and high levels of insulin start to make you gain more weight and become even more insulin resistant. It's a vicious cycle that progresses with continually rising insulin levels, greater insulin resistance, more insulin production and additional weight gain. If this cycle continues, your pancreas will ultimately fail to produce that much insulin all the time, your blood glucose will go much higher as it can't enter the cells anymore and you may need to take insulin shots (which may, unfortunately, cause you to gain more weight).

On the other hand, if you can break the cycle early by losing a good amount of weight *before* your pancreas fails to keep up with insulin demands, the chances that you can reverse your diabetes or slow its progression are high. Weight loss makes your body sensitive to insulin, which makes you like a hybrid car that needs less gasoline to function.

WHERE DOES BLOOD GLUCOSE COME FROM?

Glucose in the bloodstream comes from different sources, but the primary one is the foods you eat. Foods rich in carbohydrates (such as starches, milk, fruit and starchy root vegetables) are digested into glucose. In fact, it's normal for your blood glucose levels to modestly increase after you eat for this reason. Your body uses some glucose immediately for fuel, especially your brain, nervous system and active muscles, although all cells in the body use some glucose.

When blood glucose levels are higher (such as after a meal), extra glucose is stored in the liver and muscles as a substance called *glycogen*. When your blood glucose is low, glucagon (a hormone also made by your pancreas) tells your liver to release the stored glucose in the liver by breaking down the glycogen. When the muscles are active, they also use the glycogen already stored in the muscles to provide glucose to fuel their contractions, but that glucose doesn't leave the muscle and won't raise your blood glucose levels. Using up the glycogen in your muscles gives your body a place to easily store more carbohydrates after you eat.

HOW BLOOD GLUCOSE ENTERS CELLS AND WHY EXERCISE MATTERS

It's helpful to have a basic understanding of what is happening in your body when your glucose levels get high and what you can do about it. Regardless of whether you have prediabetes or diabetes, exercise is another way to lower insulin resistance and better manage your blood glucose levels (along with healthy eating and medications).

As mentioned earlier, the muscle cells need insulin to open the door for the glucose to enter. However, when the muscles are active during exercise it is a different story. Aside from burning calories, exercise opens the doors that allow glucose to leave your bloodstream and enter your muscle cells without the need for functional keys and keyholes. In other words, exercise bypasses the need for insulin even if you have a lot of insulin resistance at rest.

Research shows that the glucose doors will stay open for 24 to 48 hours after you're done exercising, which means that you'll continue to utilize blood glucose better during that time because your muscles need to replenish themselves and their glycogen stores. Therefore, you can help control your diabetes better by exercising at least three to four days per week. However, to lose weight most effectively, you'll likely need to aim for exercising for 60 minutes six to seven days per week.

How exercise helps insulin work (even with diabetes)

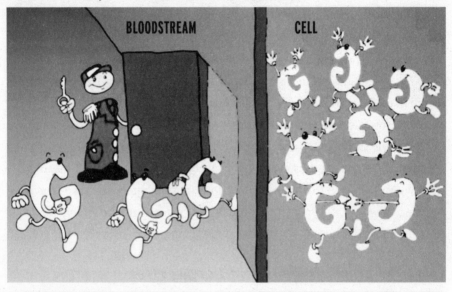

WHAT THE DIABETES BREAKTHROUGH PROGRAM CAN DO FOR YOU

While most people tend to think of managing their diabetes as a lot of deprivation, we know that isn't so. If you even make just a few of the changes in your diet that we recommend, do at least some of the physical activity you'll learn about and lose just a fraction of the extra body fat that you have, you will experience improvements in your blood glucose control and likely lower your need for diabetes medications.

How would you like to be able to reduce your insulin doses or stop taking insulin? Around 21 percent of the Why WAIT program participants who were treated with insulin stopped taking it completely by the end of the program and the rest cut their insulin doses by 50 percent or more after just 12 weeks. Taking less insulin while having good diabetes control helps in limiting future weight gain and preventing you from gaining back any weight that you lose.

Would you just like to control your diabetes on fewer daily pills? Medications are expensive and many have undesirable side effects. The majority of Why WAIT participants cut down on their diabetes pills or stopped them after a good amount of weight loss—which can also happen for you if you lose weight by following the Diabetes Breakthrough program.

What about better health? People who completed the 12-week program had sizable decreases in their blood pressure. They also saw their blood cholesterol levels improve, their kidneys work better, their risk of a heart attack get lower and their insulin action improve. In fact, two diabetes medications taken at their maximal doses can't come close to matching the effectiveness of weight loss on improving insulin action—and without any bad side effects.

What about weight loss? The majority of the Why WAIT participants have kept the weight off longer than the typical person with type 2 diabetes without the risks or the hassles associated with having to undergo gastric bypass surgery.

FIRST ACROSS THE FINISH LINE

Meet Jim. With his heart pounding, chest heaving and legs aching, Jim has never felt as alive and accomplished as the day he crossed the finish line—of his first 5K race. The 51-year-old's story starts with a bad checkup and some serious prodding by his family that convinced Jim he needed help getting his diabetes back on track.

"The doctors weren't very happy with me because of my A1C results." (In case you don't know, your A1C reflects your average blood glucose levels over the past two to three months and a number more than 7 percent indicates uncontrolled diabetes.) As Jim says, "I knew then that I'd better start making some changes if I wanted to walk my daughter down the aisle or become a grandparent." Enter the Joslin Why WAIT program and Jim's story does a U-turn to get him across that finish line, the full story of which we'll share with you later in this chapter.

ON YOUR MARK, GET SET, GO

We want to use the rest of this chapter to tell you more about what to expect from each week of this program. You will focus on different proven goals each week, but don't forget all the other ones you've already learned and started to incorporate into your life. It's the combination of all these strategies over 12 weeks that make this program the most helpful to you.

We will guide you through the process of thinking differently about your medications. You will need to work with your health care provider to strategically reduce your medications or replace those that partially contributed to your weight gain with others that help you lose weight. This is a groundbreaking concept that is unique to this program and you'll learn how to do this right from the word *go*.

The dietary plan that you will learn is easy to follow and it provides you with plenty of healthy protein and some fiber-rich carbohydrates. You will find this structured plan easy to follow, both now and for the rest of your life.

You may think you hate to exercise, but the exercise plan in this program is unlike any that you have tried (and failed doing) before. It's an innovative mix of aerobic workouts, resistance and interval training, supersets and even yoga that is enjoyable. The program will guide you slowly through it until you achieve your exercise targets of 60 minutes on most days of the week.

Finally, we don't have you set just any goals to help you succeed on this program. Instead, you'll use SMART goals (more on these later on) to learn behavioral skills that will get you safely to the finish line where you'll experience better health, a lower body weight over the long-term and renewed vigor for life.

DIABETES TAKES A MULTIFACETED APPROACH

The following triangle illustrates the eight areas of self-care important for successfully controlling your diabetes. As you can see, caring for diabetes involves finding the balance between food, exercise and medication. Recommendations for healthy eating are important, yet meal planning can be flexible and individualized. Exercise can also be tailored to meet your unique goals and needs. Diabetes medications (e.g., pills, injectable medications and insulin) are helpful for reaching your blood glucose targets. Since each person's diabetes is different, medication requirements vary. Many kinds of diabetes pills and insulin are available to help control your diabetes. It is important to find—with the help of your doctor—the right medications, especially when your body weight hangs in the balance.

Caring for Your Diabetes

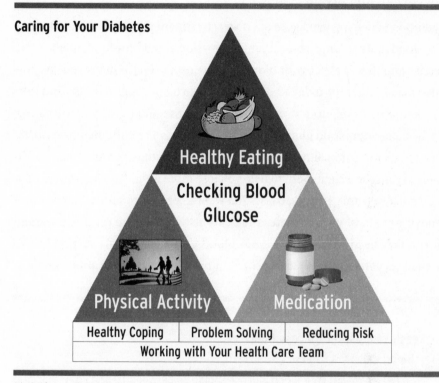

Checking blood glucose is located in the center of the triangle because it allows you to see how well these three components—food, exercise and medication—are working together to help you achieve good diabetes control. By checking frequently, you can also identify potential problems early and make changes to minimize their effect on your health and well-being.

Near the base of the triangle, the important tools of healthy coping, problem solving and reducing your risk for complications and other health problems are included. These three skills provide an important foundation that helps you to take charge of your diabetes.

Finally, at the foundation, your health care team is there to help you to learn these skills and build diabetes self-care into your life. As you start the program, we will help you make informed decisions about these areas, so you can manage your diabetes while you lose weight.

WHY CHECK YOUR BLOOD GLUCOSE?

In addition to helping you figure out if your treatment plan is working, checking your blood glucose helps you gather information about how food, medication, exercise and illness affect your blood glucose levels. It also helps you see how you're managing it from day to day and shows you patterns of highs and lows that can occur in relation to medications, exercise and foods you are eating.

Checking your blood glucose during this program can also help you realize when to talk to your health care team about making adjustments to your medication as you lose weight, both to help you lose more weight and to prevent your blood glucose from getting too low. You want to be able to reduce or eliminate some, if not all, of your diabetes medications while you're on this program, but you first need to know how your blood glucose levels are responding to the changes you're making in order to cut back on your medications safely.

Reach Your Target Glucose Goals
- Blood glucose targets
  - Before meals, your blood glucose should be between 70 and 130 mg/dl
  - If you test any time after meals, your blood glucose should be less than 180 mg/dl
  - Before you sleep, your blood glucose should be between 90 and 150 mg/dl
- A1C goal: less than 7 percent.
- Discuss your targets with your health care team.

WHAT IS YOUR A1C?

A blood test called the "A1C" represents your average blood glucose over the past two to three months. As such, the A1C is a useful indicator of what has been happening in your body over a longer period of time. Since it's an average, it doesn't tell you about the highest or lowest blood glucose levels that you have had, but research has found that an A1C below 7 percent (equivalent to average blood glucose levels of 154 mg/dl before and after meals) is best for your health now and down the road. Conversely, a blood glucose check tells you what is happening in your body right at that moment, but only at a single point in time.

It's important to know your numbers so you and your health care team can assess your overall diabetes control and help you take action as needed. Both A1C and blood glucose goals are often individualized for each person.

What Does Your A1C Equal?

A1C (percent)	AVERAGE GLUCOSE (mg/dl)	RANGE (mg/dl)
12	298	240-347
11	269	217-314
10	240	193-282
9	212	170-249
8	183	147-217
7	154	123-185
6	126	100-152
5	97	76-120

AIM FOR "A TO I" HEALTH GOALS

The ultimate aim of the weight loss that you're about to achieve is to improve your diabetes control and reduce your risk for heart disease. To effectively reach this outcome, you will need to focus on a number of health-related goals, which we have simplified by using the letters *A* to *I*:

A1C: should be lower than 7 percent
Blood Pressure: should be lower than 140/80 mmHg
Cholesterol: LDL (your bad cholesterol) should be lower than 100 mg/dl or better yet, < 70 mg/dl

Diet: follow the principles of our diet plan for life

Exercise: increase to 60 minutes most days of the week

Follow-up: follow with your diabetes health care provider every
three to six months and have your eyes checked at least every year

Glucose: your blood glucose should be 70–130 mg/dl before meals,
<180 mg/dl after meals and 90–150 mg/dl at bedtime

Happy: try to avoid stress as it raises your blood glucose and
blood pressure

I'm the one who will make all these changes.

WHY WHAT YOU EAT MATTERS

Eating a variety of food is important for good health. In this chapter, you will start to better understand how foods affect your blood glucose and weight so that you'll know how better food choices will aid both your diabetes and your weight loss efforts. In weeks to come, we will discuss appropriate serving and portion sizes and how they fit into your meal plan. We'll also explain why you should start by using meal replacements for breakfast and lunch for at least the first six weeks you're on the program.

By the end of 12 weeks, we expect that your attitude toward food may have changed greatly. In fact, we will teach you how to make healthy food choices without feeling restricted or deprived and how to eat well for both diabetes and weight management. Implementing these changes in attitudes and behaviors takes time, but by the end of this program, you'll be armed with the knowledge, strategies and support that you need to succeed at managing your diabetes and your weight for a long and healthy life.

WHERE DO CALORIES COME FROM?

All three major nutrients coming from foods and drinks—carbohydrate, protein and fat, otherwise known as macronutrients—contain calories and so does alcohol. Often in diabetes, we get very focused on carbohydrate-rich foods and forget that while carbohydrates are the main nutrient affecting blood glucose, calories are what affect your body weight. Since all the macronutrients contain calories, you also need to be mindful of protein- and fat-rich foods that may or may not have many carbohydrates in them to achieve your weight loss goals.

Many people think that carbohydrates have more calories than protein, but they actually have the same number of calories per gram (four). At nine, fat has more than twice as many calories per gram, which is why you need to watch your serving sizes of fats. High-fat foods can add up quickly when it comes to calories. For instance, just a small handful of nuts has around 180 calories. Just think how easy it is to eat many handfuls of nuts without even thinking about it. Moderation is the key when it comes to eating higher calorie foods.

Calories Come From

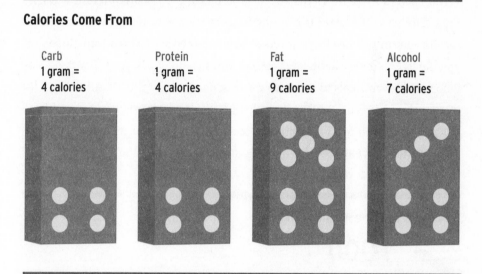

Carb	Protein	Fat	Alcohol
1 gram =	1 gram =	1 gram =	1 gram =
4 calories	4 calories	9 calories	7 calories

It's also important to consider your alcohol choices as part of your total calories. Alcohol is a source of pure calories (seven calories per gram, almost as much as fat) without any other nutrients like vitamins and minerals. If you drink any alcohol, be sure to factor the calories into your meal plan that come from both the alcohol itself and any mixers or residual sugars. Although wine and alcohol in general may have some heart health benefits, it is recommended that women should not exceed one (five-ounce) glass of wine or other drink per day and men no more than two drinks.

HOW FOODS AFFECT YOUR BLOOD GLUCOSE

As mentioned, the three major macronutrients are carbohydrate, protein and fat. They supply your body with energy or calories, although each of these nutrients has a different primary role. Protein helps to build muscle, while fat is important as a source of stored energy as well as for the health of your brain, nerves, hair, skin and nails. Carbohydrate is a major fuel source for your body, especially during physical activity and is the primary supplier of energy for your brain, nerves and muscles.

Do you know which food category affects your blood glucose the most? While each of these nutrients affects your blood glucose in different ways, it's important to realize that the carbohydrates you eat have the greatest impact on the amount of glucose in your blood because they are turned into glucose as you digest them very soon after eating. You should check your blood glucose before and after meals to learn how foods, particularly those containing a lot of carbohydrate (such as potatoes, bread, rice and pasta), affect your blood glucose. Only minimal amounts of protein and fat become glucose after digestion, so they don't affect your blood glucose nearly as much.

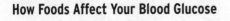

How Foods Affect Your Blood Glucose

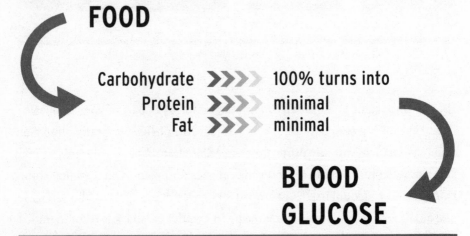

FOOD

Carbohydrate	⟫⟫	100% turns into
Protein	⟫⟫	minimal
Fat	⟫⟫	minimal

BLOOD GLUCOSE

DIGESTION OF FOOD CAN BE TIME-DELAYED

Your blood glucose is at its highest generally one hour after eating, remains high for up to two hours and then starts to fall. Have you noticed this happening after you eat a meal? Check your blood glucose two hours after you eat to obtain a picture of how the carbohydrate foods you eat affect your blood glucose. When you eat a higher fat meal, your digestive process (otherwise known as *gastric emptying*) is slowed down and your blood glucose may not reach its highest point two hours after eating, but rather four to six hours later. What's more, high-fat foods cause insulin resistance which, together with slower digestion, may lead to higher blood glucose levels hours after you eat them when your muscle, fat and liver cells are not using the insulin in your body properly to lower blood glucose. Examples of higher fat meals are macaroni and cheese, fettuccine Alfredo pasta, fried foods and pizza. Many of these are best considered "get you now, get you later" foods because of their dual effects on raising your blood glucose.

Gastric Emptying (assuming a low fat meal)

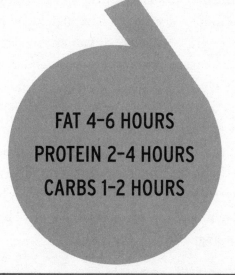

FAT 4–6 HOURS

PROTEIN 2–4 HOURS

CARBS 1–2 HOURS

CALORIES IN, CALORIES OUT

Achieving and maintaining a healthy weight is a balancing act of "calories in" and "calories out." We have just begun to discuss the calories that you take in from the foods you eat. To successfully lose weight, it isn't enough to just limit your calorie intake; you also need to burn calories through physical activity, which is one of the many reasons for the exercise component of the Diabetes Breakthrough program. In future chapters, we will discuss strategies that will help you find this balance and practice the skills needed to reach your weight loss goal while managing your diabetes.

DO YOU NEED TO GET A CHECKUP FIRST?

Depending on your age, your general health and your physical activity level, you may need to consider getting a checkup from your health care team before starting our (or any other) structured exercise program. At the checkup, get your blood pressure, heart rate and body weight checked and ask whether you need to do an exercise stress test, which usually involves walking on a treadmill or riding a stationary bike for around ten minutes.

An exercise stress test is only recommended by the American Diabetes Association if you're over 40 and have diabetes or if you're over 30, have had diabetes for 10 or more years, smoke, have high blood pressure, have high blood cholesterol levels, or have eye or kidney problems related to diabetes—but *only* if you're planning to do vigorous training that gets your heart rate up really high. If you'll just be doing moderate aerobic activity and mild resistance training, such extensive (and often expensive) testing may not be necessary for anyone who is reasonably healthy.

If you're already very active, getting an extra checkup before you replace your current exercise regime with the program's exercise routine is definitely not necessary. If you have any concerns, check with your health care provider at your next visit to discuss any precautions that may be important for your health when exercising.

START BEING MORE PHYSICALLY ACTIVE

It's never too late to regain a great deal of the physical fitness you have lost by being physically inactive. What's more, regular exercise can also improve your coordination, balance and posture. If you're already over 40 years old and haven't started exercising yet, now is definitely the time to begin. A recent study on exercise demonstrated that even for people who are already middle-aged, exercising more can add years to their lives and you can be assured that those extra years are much more likely to be lived well—which is even more critical when you have a chronic health condition like diabetes.

Your home exercise program will primarily consist of a combination of aerobic, resistance and flexibility exercises. You'll progress gradually from doing 20 minutes of exercise four days per week up to 60 minutes of exercise six days per week (continuous or intermittent), which is overviewed in the 12-week exercise progression table.

Every day you do some planned exercise (four to six days per week), you will include some aerobic activity. Starting about the third or fourth week of the program, you'll also be substituting in some resistance training for part of your training time two to three nonconsecutive days per week. Every day you exercise you should do some stretching, but that particular activity counts minimally toward the total time for each day or the week. The total amount of time you spend exercising—regardless of whether it's aerobic, resistance, circuit, interval, superset or other training—adds toward your daily and weekly exercise goals.

Diabetes Breakthrough 12-Week Exercise Plan Overview

WEEK	EXERCISE	DURATION	FREQUENCY	TYPES OF EXERCISE
1	Aerobic	17 minutes	4 days	Aerobic
	Stretching	3 minutes	4 days	Stretching
		20 minutes total		
2	Aerobic	22 minutes	4 days	Aerobic
	Stretching	3 minutes	4 days	Cross training
		25 minutes total		Stretching

continued

WEEK	EXERCISE	DURATION	FREQUENCY	TYPES OF EXERCISE
3	Aerobic	17* to 27** minutes	4 days	Aerobic
	Resistance	10 minutes	2 days	Resistance
	Stretching	3 minutes	4 days	training
		30 minutes total		Stretching
4	Aerobic	22* to 37** minutes	4 days	Aerobic
	Resistance	15 minutes	2 days	Circuit training
	Stretching	3 minutes	4 days	Cross training
		40 minutes total		Stretching
5	Aerobic	12* to 37** minutes	5 days	Interval training
	Resistance	25 minutes	3 days	Resistance
	Stretching	3 minutes	5 days	training
		40 minutes total		Stretching
6	Aerobic	16* to 41** minutes	5 days	Interval training
	Resistance	25 minutes	3 days	Core stability
	Stretching	4 minutes	5 days	training
		45 minutes total		Yoga
				Stretching
7	Aerobic	11* to 41** minutes	5 days	Interval training
	Resistance	30 minutes	3 days	Superset training
	Stretching	4 minutes	5 days	Stretching
		45 minutes total		
8	Aerobic	11* to 46** minutes	5 days	Interval training
	Resistance	35 minutes	3 days	Circuit training
	Stretching	4 minutes	5 days	Stretching
		50 minutes total		
9	Aerobic	10* to 50** minutes	6 days	Interval training
	Resistance	40 minutes	3 days	Superset training
	Stretching	5 minutes	6 days	Stretching
		55 minutes total		

10	Aerobic	15* to 55** minutes	6 days	Interval training
	Resistance	40 minutes	3 days	Core stability
	Stretching	5 minutes	6 days	training
		60 minutes total		Yoga
				Stretching
11-12	Aerobic	15* to 55** minutes	6 days	Interval training
	Resistance	40 minutes	3 days	Superset training
	Stretching	5 minutes	6 days	Stretching
		60 minutes total		

* Minutes of aerobic exercise on days including resistance training.
** Minutes of aerobic exercise on days without resistance training.

Although doing the planned activities that we recommend is critical to your long-term weight loss success, increasing your daily movement is equally as important to losing weight as it is to keeping it off. You may only exercise for an hour most days of the week, but that leaves 23 hours of every day when you can burn off even more calories just by moving more. Standing, fidgeting and walking anywhere can add up to 350 extra burned calories by the end of each day and a whole lot over time.

LEARN TO BE SMART

The Diabetes Breakthrough program features the use of SMART goals to get you motivated, determine where you want to be headed and help keep you on the right path. Diabetes and body weight are challenges that are here for life, so you need to start thinking more about what behavioral changes you think you can establish and maintain as a new habit for a lifetime.

The SMART goals that you will be using work as follows:

- **S** stands for **Specific**
  For example, you could say, "I want to eat better." Or you can set a SMART goal like this one: "I will eat two servings of vegetables at every meal." Which one are you more likely to do? (Hint: Just pick the veggies you really like.)

- **M** means **Measurable**

  How many times have you promised yourself already that you're going to exercise more—and how many times have you failed at doing just that? It's time for a measurable goal like "I will exercise for 30 minutes a day, five days a week," which you will put on your daily schedule to make it a priority.

- **A** stands for **Action-oriented**

  What do you think an action-oriented goal would involve? Should you make a promise to *(a)* "Drink some soda *after* I realize my blood glucose is low following exercise because I started feeling symptoms" or *(b)* "Check my blood glucose before and after exercise and treat any lows by eating some of the glucose tablets I carry in my purse"? If you answered *(b)*, then you're already getting SMARTer.

- **R** reminds you to be **Realistic**

  While you may want to lose 50 pounds in two months (like grocery store magazines promise), a more realistic goal would be: "I will work on losing one to two pounds a week until I reach my weight goal." The Diabetes Breakthrough program's SMART steps are designed to make that happen.

- **T** says to make your goals **Time-limited**

  If you promise to "increase my exercise time as I get more fit," you're apt to fail. How about making this promise instead? "I'll add five minutes to each of my walks this week." Another component of a time-limited goal is to establish a time to reassess your progress toward your goals.

TAKE THE TIME TO BE SMART

How many times have you been told by a health care provider that you really need to lose weight and exercise more? If you said "zero," we would be really shocked. When you were given this advice, what did it really mean to you? It's kind of vague when you think about it. What exactly does "lose weight" mean? Twenty pounds or 100? In the next two months or over the next year? How exactly will you accomplish this goal? What will you eat and what will you do for exercise? Here's where setting SMART goals comes in. They help you set goals in a systematic and focused way.

As you just read, SMART goals are Specific, Measurable, Action-oriented, Realistic and Time-limited. To turn this vague advice into a tangible goal, ask yourself the following questions: How much weight am I planning to lose, in what time frame and using what strategies and approaches to meal planning? With regard to exercise, what types of exercise will I do, when will I schedule it and for how long and how often per week will I do it? While the goals for your first month on the program will actually be defined for you by the Diabetes Breakthrough meal plan and exercise plan, you still need to be able to set workable goals for the rest of your life. Now is as good a time as any to begin thinking in this new mode so that you can use SMART goal-setting as a tool to keep you going after the program ends.

Before you move forward to the first week of the program, practice setting at least two SMART goals, one in each of the areas listed (i.e., nutrition and physical activity). In addition, list what you think your barriers to achieving each goal may be and an action plan for overcoming them. Anticipating potential barriers to meeting your goals and developing a plan in advance for overcoming these barriers will aid you with successfully losing weight and keeping it off for good. Be certain to revisit your goals every week, evaluate how well they worked, update them as needed and congratulate yourself on the ones you have achieved.

Here are some examples of vague versus SMART goals to get you started.

Not specific: *I will eat better.*
Specific: *I will eat two servings of vegetables at every meal.*
Not measurable: *I will exercise more.*
Measurable: *I will exercise for 30 minutes a day five days a week.*
Not action-oriented: *I'll know if my blood glucose is low after I exercise if I start feeling symptoms and then I'll drink some soda.*
Action-oriented: *I will check my blood glucose before/after exercise and treat any lows by taking the glucose tabs that I carry in my purse.*
Not realistic: *I will lose 50 pounds in two months.*
Realistic: *I will lose one to two pounds a week.*

Not time-limited: *I'll increase my exercise time as I get more fit.*
Time-limited: *I'll add five minutes to each of my walks this week. I'll evaluate my progress at the end of the week and may even set a new goal.*

List Two SMART Goals You Will Work on for the Upcoming Month:

NUTRITION/DIET

I will: _____

_____

Potential barriers: _____

_____

Action plan for overcoming barriers: _____

_____

Evaluation: What worked? What didn't work?_____

_____

_____

PHYSICAL ACTIVITY/EXERCISE

I will: _____

_____

Potential barriers: _____

_____

Action plan for overcoming barriers: _____

_____

Evaluation: What worked? What didn't work?_____

_____

_____

GET EQUIPPED WITH SUPPLIES FOR SUCCESS

Although we certainly do not require you to buy anything to follow this program, we do suggest buying, borrowing or making what you already have work for the following items:

- **Measuring cups and spoons:** Any kitchen variety will do, but make sure to have at least a set of ¼, ⅓, ½ and 1 cup measures to use, along with teaspoon and tablespoon measuring spoons.
- **Kitchen scale:** A number of scales are available that will measure ounces and grams for you; pick up an inexpensive one of those to use.
- **Resistance bands (three different tensions, with door anchor):** You can pick up an inexpensive set of three bands at any sporting goods store, but also at places like Target®, Walmart®, some clothing stores and online at Amazon (such as Black Mountain Products Resistance Band Set with Door Anchor) and elsewhere. Try to get a package of three resistance bands (light, moderate and high intensity) with a door anchor; handles are recommended for a better grip and easier use.
- **Comfortable workout clothes:** A pair of shorts and a T-shirt, yoga pants or sweats work well—loose-fitting clothing is more comfortable—although anything that allows your free range of motion around all joints is acceptable.
- **Appropriate shoes for exercise:** You want to make sure to have some athletic or custom shoes that fit well and are not likely to cause blisters. Check your feet daily after wear, though, just to check for problem areas. Also, replace walking shoes at least every six months to reduce the stress on your knees and other lower body joints.
- **Blood glucose meter and test strips:** For this program, we recommend that you check your blood glucose levels more frequently than normal—at least four to six times a day to start—to learn the effects of your lifestyle improvements on your diabetes control, to detect low blood glucose and to help

determine when you may need to consult with your health care provider about lowering your medication doses or eliminating some of them.

- **Notebook for logbook:** We provide you with a prototype logbook for menus and exercise training. You can copy and paste those into a notebook or just set up your own way to record your various values.

- **Sense of humor:** While not critical to losing weight, being able to laugh does help lower your cortisol levels, which can make it easier for you to lower your insulin needs and to lose weight.

"Oh, My Aching Feet"

You may have flat feet, high arches, wide feet or joint problems that can exacerbate if you do not wear the proper footwear. Many people with diabetes tend to have flat feet from the extra body weight that they have, which could lead to joint and muscle pain. Shoes with more stability like cross-training athletic ones provide more arch support and reduce risk of injuries and custom orthotics may also be beneficial for some people. Talk with your health care provider or a podiatrist (foot doctor) to find out what may be the proper footwear for your unique feet. In addition, many stores specialize in matching you with the right shoes for your feet.

RACE TO A HEALTHIER LIFE

Remember Jim, the runner from the beginning of this chapter? He not only reached the average goals of the Why WAIT program, but he also vastly exceeded them. By the end of the 12 weeks, he had shed 40 pounds and soon thereafter dropped his blood glucose into a normal range—despite having been taken off all of his diabetes medications *and* one for high blood pressure.

When he started the program his goal was to run a 5K (5 kilometer or 3.1 mile) race. He hasn't just met that goal; he has since participated in other 5K and 10K (6.2 mile) races and has consistently placed first or second in his age group. What's more, he is currently training for a half marathon that he plans to run with his oldest son this year. Now that's an example of a well-defined SMART goal.

How did he do it? Jim says, "Determination is what it finally took for me to make these changes in my lifestyle for the better. I am now more determined than ever to stay on my path to keep myself healthier." Diabetes can lead you across the finish line, too—and to a healthier and longer life in the process—even if you don't take up running road races.

DIABETES BREAKTHROUGH WEEK 1

Meal Plans, Logbooks, Exercise Barriers and Stretching

This first official week of the Diabetes Breakthrough program starts with a weigh-in, learning how to plan your meals (including the choice of using tasty shakes for breakfast and lunch), figuring out what's keeping you from exercising, beginning easy aerobic exercise workouts and using a logbook to record your blood glucose levels, diet, exercise and challenges. You have your work cut out for you.

This week is a preview of all to come, but an important one for assembling all the tools you'll need going forward with the rest of the program. Your success from one week builds on the next one and each week you should be seeing some progress and know even more about what it takes to lose the weight and keep it off for good—all while controlling your blood glucose levels better than ever. While we'll revisit some topics from time to time, always feel free to go back and reread a previous chapter or two for ideas or inspiration.

PRAYING FOR THE HELP THE PROGRAM BROUGHT HER

For some people, finding your way is a spiritual experience. For Donna, who just turned 60, the Joslin Why WAIT program was literally the answer to her prayers. She'd been having lots of problems with her diabetes and had been praying about what to do. When she met with Dr. Hamdy, he convinced her to give the Why WAIT program a try. She recalls, "I was afraid. I thought I couldn't exercise because of my arthritic knees." Boy, was she ever surprised when she was both able to exercise and reach all her weight loss and blood glucose goals. We'll tell you a little later how well it has worked for her.

WEIGH IN, MEASURE UP, PICK A PAIR AND WALK A BIT

It's always good to have a starting place—that way you can easily tell when you've improved and how much. We'd like you to take some baseline measurements that you can repeat at the end of 12 weeks to measure your progress. Try the following this week:

- **Weigh in:** This first week of the program requires you to weigh yourself on a scale and record your starting weight. In order to know in real terms how well the program is working for you, it's important that you establish your starting point. Knowing that will also help you begin to set realistic weight loss goals. Only weigh yourself one time a week and always make sure you're weighing in at the same time of day under similar circumstances (e.g., after your morning shower, without clothes or with the same minimal clothing on and before eating breakfast).

- **Measure up:** If you have access to a tape measure, now is also a good time to have someone help you measure your waist (at the level of your natural waist or about one inch above your belly button), your hips (at their widest point) and even your upper arm or anywhere else you expect to be losing some inches. If nothing else, it will be motivating for you to see how many inches you've dropped from different areas. (If you have access to a machine that measures body fat, feel free to measure that as well now and then again in 12 weeks.)

- **Pick a pair:** Of course, you can always just use the good old clothes test. Pick one pair of pants that you can currently fit into (even if you have to hold your breath to get them on)—preferably ones that do not have an elastic waist—and see how well they fit or don't fit you now. Use the same pair of pants as your point of reference. As you start to lose weight and inches from around your waist, hips and thighs, you should be able to tell when they are starting to fit you better (or get too big for the new, improved you).

- **Walk a bit:** This measure of your current fitness involves doing a six-minute walk test, a timed test to see how far you can walk in six minutes. For this test, walk as far as you can in six minutes at a pace that does not cause pain. If you have access to a treadmill, you can measure the distance you cover in that amount of time on that, but otherwise simply set out from your house (and follow the same path later with your car) or go to a track to find out the distance you can travel in that amount of time. When you revisit this test after 12 weeks, if you use the same path or testing mode, you'll be able to see your improvement very clearly.

GET READY FOR BLOOD GLUCOSE CHECKING

During the first month or so of this program, you'll need to check your blood glucose levels more often than usual—at least four to six times per day, including before (and sometimes two to three hours after) each meal, before and after exercise and at bedtime—so you can work with your health care provider to lower your medications safely and effectively to prevent low blood glucose (a reading <70 mg/dl) that can happen when your extra pounds start to drop off. After the first month, you may still want to check more frequently, but it's not quite as critical as it is during the start of the program when you're more likely to need bigger adjustments to your medications. We prefer that you use one of the glucose meters that keep an electronic log of blood glucose and activity. In the Why WAIT program, we use the Lifescan One Touch® or the Abbott FreeStyle® meters since they are covered by most insurance plans and data can easily be downloaded from them.

HOW PEOPLE GET "PORTION DISTORTION"

In this chapter, we're going to start talking about portions and serving sizes and continue that over the next few weeks. Portion control is a crucial aspect of healthy eating. Although no food is really "bad," some foods are best when eaten only in small quantities. However, many people experience "portion distortion" and are confused about what an appropriate portion size is. You'll find some handy references for estimating portion sizes in subsequent chapters.

First, let's discuss the difference between a portion size and a serving size. People tend to interpret the size of their meal, regardless of how big or small it may be, to be an appropriate portion. But a "serving" isn't the amount you put on your plate: it's a specific amount of food, defined by common measurements such as cups, ounces or pieces. You'll find serving sizes listed on food labels. A "portion" is the amount of a food that you choose to eat and can be more or less than a serving.

If you eat a small snack pack of Ritz Bits®, for example, you may consider that your serving. However, if you have a large box in front of you, you may eat the whole box and consider *that* your serving. A box of Ritz Bits® actually contains several servings. That's why smaller packages, such as 100-calorie snack packs, have been hugely successful since they have portion control built right in.

Portion Size Versus Serving Size
- Many people think the portion in front of them is the appropriate portion size to eat.
- A serving size is a determined amount on a food label and may or may not be the correct portion size.
- What is an appropriate portion size varies from person to person.

Let's look at another example. The serving size listed on the back of a box of Teddy Grahams® is 10. The nutrition information listed on the back of the box relates to the same 10 Teddy Grahams®. What if you decide to eat 20 of them because 10 just didn't fill you up? Your portion then becomes two servings, so you need to double the content for all of the nutrients, such as calories, carbohydrates and fats.

In one study done on portion sizes, researchers gave participants a lunch of macaroni and cheese every day. Each day, they were unknowingly served larger and larger amounts of macaroni and cheese. The participants ate everything they were served; they didn't realize that they were actually eating more each day. In another study, researchers examined this issue by comparing the calories consumed by a group served soup from a standard soup bowl with others eating from a soup bowl that was secretly being refilled. Participants who ate from the refilling bowls ate 73 percent more soup, but reported feeling no more satiated than those who didn't.

Really, most people don't conceptualize portion sizes very well or have a good sense of their hunger or satiety. Remember, however, that an appropriate portion size is different for everyone. Those of you on the 1200-calorie meal plan for this program will eat a different portion of rice than what's recommended for the people on the 1800-calorie plan.

To be successful using your Diabetes Breakthrough meal plan, it's important that you learn what portions and what types of foods you're supposed to have. You'll need to decide on exactly which foods and how much of them you are going to have and then buy them.

WHY CALORIES MATTER

Your diet and exercise patterns dramatically impact how much body fat you have. Of course, this is not news. How you gain and lose weight can affect your body fat levels as well. For example, most people who diet lose both fat and muscle and when they regain the weight, they gain back fat—ending up fatter than before they lost weight. Not so for the Why WAIT participants: In 2013, over 500 participants had lost an average of 24 pounds after only 12 weeks, while gaining muscle mass, meaning that they lost fat at a healthy rate (unlike most fad diets) and none of their precious muscle.

How did you gain weight in the first place? Well, larger portions contain more calories. Being physically inactive is also a contributing factor since being more active burns more daily calories. Calories are the fuel needed to keep our bodies functioning at rest, during our day-to-day activities and when we're exercising. Each of us requires a certain number of calories each day to maintain our current weight. Generally speaking, if you eat more than what your body needs, you'll gain weight and if you eat less, you'll lose weight.

While weight loss may slow down over time, cutting out 500 calories a day from your diet can result in a weight loss of one pound per week. Although it can vary by the body tissue, there are approximately 3500 calories in a pound of body fat. To gain a pound, you need to eat at least that many calories more than your body requires for maintenance. To lose a pound, you need to eat that much less, or you can burn more calories through physical activity. Most likely, you would need to cut out 500 calories a day to lose about a pound in a week (7 days x 500 calories = 3500 calories = 1 pound), but weight loss can vary based on a number of other factors, as discussed below.

Calories and Pounds of Body Fat
- There are approximately 3500 calories in a pound.
- Cut out 500 calories a day to lose about a pound a week.
- This calorie reduction can add up to a smaller you over time.

HOW MUCH WEIGHT WILL YOU LOSE (AND WHEN)?

During the first week or two of a diet, it's possible and pretty common to lose a lot more than a pound—up to as much as eight to ten pounds per week. The reason is that you lose more water weight at first (stored with carbohydrates in muscles) when you first cut back on calories and start being more active. Rapid weight loss is almost always mostly water weight (from muscle) and very temporary. After the first couple of weeks, however, what you're losing should be mostly fat weight and that contains more calories per pound than other tissues.

When you exercise while cutting back on calories, that can also slow down your weight loss on the scale because muscle (which you're gaining or retaining) adds to your overall weight even as you lose body fat—and the result is a slower change on the scale. Keeping your muscle mass is essential to keeping the weight off for good, though, so don't despair if you're not losing weight as fast as you think you should.

We said that cutting back by 3500 calories usually allows you to lose a pound of fat per week, but that is not always the case. For instance, a recent study in *Lancet* showed that estimating the energy content of weight lost as 3500 calories per pound ignores how your body is adapting to its new (lower) body weight. Both your resting metabolism (the calories you burn while sleeping or during rest) and how many calories you use doing exercise decrease as you lose weight (especially if you lose muscle mass). Your body has to make these adaptations to survive since you can't lose a pound a week indefinitely. If a 300-pound dieter could really lose a pound a week by cutting his or her regular diet by 500 calories a day, that person would vanish entirely in six years. A more realistic formula is that this caloric reduction would lead you to lose 50 pounds over three or more years.

WHAT WILL YOU BE EATING?

Dieting has never been so easy. To lose weight on this program, you will be cutting back on your daily calories while adding in more exercise and other healthy lifestyle behaviors. Your healthy diet will include approximately 40–45 percent of your daily calories coming from carbohydrates, 20–30 percent from protein and 30–35 percent from fat. The meal plan is especially designed to help you work toward your diabetes and weight loss goals. It gives you the right macronutrient distribution for meals that will help you lose weight and keep your blood glucose levels in good control. Even though the meal plan is already designed and is in a cookie-cutter format, you will learn in the next 12 weeks how to create your own menus and how to balance a meal appropriately when dining away from home.

"What's for Dinner?"

For your convenience, food choices, ideas, recipes with exact calorie counts and menus for all three meals have been included in this book. Look for them in the following places:

- Breakfast menu choices and examples: Appendix A
- Lunch menu exchanges and 12 recipes: Appendix B
- Dinner menu exchanges, 17 recipes each for 1200, 1500 and 1800 calories and acceptable frozen dinner meals (listed by brand): Appendix C
- Joslin Diabetes Center Nutritional Guidelines: Appendix D

This dietary plan is based on research showing how to best manage blood glucose levels and simplify weight loss. Carbohydrates have the biggest impact on blood glucose control and, therefore, they are limited to 40–45 percent of calories. The carbohydrate choices that are included in the meal plan are mostly high-fiber ones, which should help in keeping you satisfied after meals and control your postmeal blood glucose spikes. Protein accounts for 20–30 percent of your total calories and will help maintain your muscle, keep you feeling fuller and hold your blood glucose levels in check, particularly since you will be picking healthy sources of protein. Fat accounts for 30–35 percent of your calories to supply your body with healthy, essential fats. Fat choices included in the meal plan are heart-healthy fats and include no unnatural trans fats; your saturated fat intake will also not exceed 7 percent of total calories as many of those fats coming from processed meats and dairy may raise your bad cholesterol levels.

EAT MORE PROTEIN

The increased amount of protein in the plan is a critical part of why this menu is so effective for losing weight and managing your diabetes. Protein has a minimal effect on blood glucose levels and it aids in the sensation of fullness. In fact, low-protein meal plans are associated with increased hunger. Thus, eating more lean protein together with healthy fats may serve to reduce your appetite and help you to achieve and maintain a lower calorie level. As mentioned, adequate intake of protein also helps to maintain lean body mass (muscle mass) during weight reduction so that you primarily lose body fat— and this is key to helping you keep off the weight you lose.

Recommended healthy protein sources include fish, skinless poultry, nonfat or low-fat dairy, eggs and egg whites, tofu, tempeh and seitan. However, you should not increase your protein intake from high saturated fat animal sources (e.g., beef, pork, lamb and high-fat dairy products), as those may be associated with an increased risk for heart attack and stroke.

On the flip side, a recent study in the *Journal of the American Medical Association* showed that weight gain caused by eating 1000 extra calories a day is also affected by how much protein you eat. People on a low-protein diet gain less extra weight overall, but what they gain is all fat since they lose muscle due to being protein deficient. That's not a pretty picture, either.

Does Your Plate Look like This?

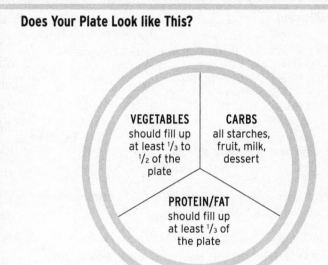

- Is your plate covered with colorful vegetables: dark green, orange, red and yellow?
- Is the fat trimmed off your meat and skin taken off?
- Did you choose leaner cuts of meat, poultry or fish?
- Did you choose whole grain pasta or breads? Brown rice or potato with skin?
- How much fat was used in cooking or added to your plate?
- Did you boil, steam, grill or bake instead of frying your foods?

CHOOSE THE RIGHT CALORIE PLAN FOR YOU

On this program, you will be following a meal plan that has either 1500 calories or 1800 calories a day. Regardless of your recommended total calories, the Diabetes Breakthrough meal plan recommends a balance of carbohydrates, protein and fat, as previously discussed.

Due to differences in body size and composition, most *women* should start out following our *1500-calorie plan*. The calories are distributed among three meals and two or three daily snacks.

1500-Calorie Plan (Women)

BREAKFAST	Diabetes-friendly meal replacement shake (to start): Ultra Glucose Control®, Boost Glucose Control®, Boost Calorie Smart® or Glucerna Hunger Smart®	190 calories
LUNCH	Meal replacement shake (to start), plus 1 vegetable serving and 1 fat serving	190 + 50 + 100 calories
DINNER	60 grams carbs, 45 grams protein (6 ounces) and 20 grams fat (approximately)	600 calories
SNACKS	2-3 snacks throughout the day	400 calories total
TOTAL	All meals	~1530 calories

Most *men* should start out on the *1800-calorie plan*. If you do and find that you're not losing your goal of one pound per week, cut back to the 1500-calorie plan for a week or two to see if that helps. (Also, check your actual portion sizes using measuring cups or a kitchen scale.)

1800-Calorie Plan (Men)

BREAKFAST	Diabetes-friendly meal replacement shake (to start): Ultra Glucose Control®, Boost Glucose Control®, Boost Calorie Smart® or Glucerna Hunger Smart®	190 calories
LUNCH	Meal replacement shake (to start), plus 1 vegetable serving, 2 fat servings and 1 fruit serving	190 + 50 + 200 + 60 calories

DINNER	70 grams carbs, 52.5 grams protein (7.5 ounces) and 23 grams fat (approximately)	700 calories
SNACKS	2-3 snacks throughout the day	400 calories total
TOTAL	All meals	~1790 calories

For anyone starting out on the 1500-calorie plan who is not successfully losing weight, he or she may want to switch to the 1200-calorie plan, but this is *not* a recommended menu plan on which anyone (female or male) should start. Snacks for this menu only total 300 calories, but can be added onto meals instead if preferred.

1200-Calorie Plan

BREAKFAST	Diabetes-friendly meal replacement shake (to start): Ultra Glucose Control®, Boost Glucose Control®, Boost Calorie Smart® or Glucerna Hunger Smart®	190 calories
LUNCH	Meal replacement shake (to start), plus 1 vegetable serving and 1 fat serving	190 + 50 + 100 calories
DINNER	50 grams carbs, 37.5 grams protein (5 ounces) and 17 grams fat (approximately)	500 calories
SNACKS	1-3 snacks throughout the day	300 calories total
TOTAL	All meals	~1330 calories

Your Diabetes Breakthrough Meal Plan:
- Based on 40-45 percent of total daily calories from carbohydrate, 20-30 percent from protein and 30-35 percent fat.
- Set at 1500 or 1800 daily calories to start for most women and men, respectively.
- Uses meal replacement shakes to reduce food choices and aid in calorie control (at least for the first six weeks).
- High in fiber to promote fullness (and good health).

USE MEAL REPLACEMENT SHAKES

We strongly recommend using meal replacement shakes as they aid in calorie control by reducing food choices while their high-fiber, protein and fat content help you to feel full. The Diabetes Breakthrough plan includes using them at breakfast and at lunch for *at least the first six weeks* of the program.

When picking meal replacement shakes, choose from any of the three diabetes-friendly ones that we currently recommend to our participants that follow the same dietary composition ratio of the Why WAIT meal plans:

- Ultra Glucose Control®
- Boost Glucose Control®
- Boost Calorie Smart®
- Glucerna Hunger Smart

With under 200 calories each, all of these shakes are made specifically for weight management and they optimize blood glucose control, as well. You can purchase them at stores like CVS®, Walgreens®, Walmart®, Kmart® and Target® (among others) and many places online. Using an equivalent store brand that saves you money is also acceptable as long as the one you choose has a similar number of calories and carbohydrates. (Ensure® has too many carbohydrates to be equivalent.)

If you find that these shakes are no longer as enjoyable as they were at the start, feel free to jazz them up a bit. For example, you can mix your shakes with coffee, add them to club soda and drink them through a straw, or put them in a wineglass.

Meal replacement shakes limit choice, provide structure and fit the nutrient profile of the program's meals and snacks. They also help with fullness and blood glucose control, but keep in mind that they are a tool, not a permanent replacement, for breakfast and lunch. Breakfast and lunch menus are included in Appendix A and Appendix B to replace the shakes during the program (usually after the first six weeks) and you are highly encouraged to practice eating "real food" as well since this is your goal for long-term meal planning.

Be aware that blood glucose patterns frequently change when you start using meal replacements and your diabetes medications may need adjustment to prevent low blood glucose. Talk to your health care provider about modifying your doses if you find yourself developing any low blood glucose levels related to this change in your dietary patterns.

CHOOSE YOUR FOODS WISELY

See the lists that follow for food options (vegetable, fat, fruit and snack servings) and serving sizes. Sample breakfast, lunch and dinner menus can be found in Appendices A, B and C, respectively. In addition, an overview of the Joslin Diabetes Center's nutritional guidelines on which this program's meal plans are based is in Appendix D.

If you aren't able to cook your own meals or don't like to, it is possible to use some frozen meals to meet your suggested calorie intake for dinner in particular (usually 600–700 calories, depending on your appropriate meal plan), which are included in Appendix C with the dinner recipes. Many of the Lean Cuisine®, Healthy Choice® and Smart Ones® frozen dinners meet the recommended amounts of carbohydrates, fat and protein as well as calories. Oftentimes you will get to eat two frozen meals to reach your calorie goals. If you find that you cannot finish dinners and you choose to eat only one, you can add another 200-calorie snack at some other time of day as needed.

Vegetable Servings

Feel free to snack on any of the vegetables on this list when hungry. A *serving* is the equivalent of *1 cup raw* and *½ cup cooked* veggies, both of which contain five grams of carbohydrate. An insulin bolus (if you take insulin) may be needed to cover some veggies.

- Lettuce
- Tomatoes
- Carrots
- Spinach
- Cucumbers
- Onions
- Mushrooms
- Broccoli
- Cauliflower
- Kale
- Collard greens
- String/green beans
- Asparagus
- Artichoke hearts
- Bell peppers
- Brussels sprouts
- Cabbage
- Celery
- Zucchini/ summer squash
- Eggplants
- Radishes
- Beets
- Water chestnuts

Fat Servings

Choose one serving from this list to use with veggies at lunch (1200- and 1500-calorie plans). Choose two servings on the 1800-calorie plan.

- 1 tablespoon peanut butter
- ⅛ cup any nut
- 1½ tablespoon regular salad dressing
- 2 tablespoons seeds
- 2 tablespoons light dressing
- 1 tablespoon oil
- 2 slices 2% milk or low-fat cheese
- 1 slice full-fat cheese
- 2 light string cheeses or 1 regular string cheese
- ¼ cup shredded cheese
- ½ cup low-fat cottage cheese

Fruit Servings

A *serving* of fruit contains *15 grams of carbohydrate* and *60 calories.* Pick from the following for lunch only if on the 1800-calorie menu plan, or use as snacks on other plans.

- Apple (4 ounces)
- Banana (4 ounces, ½ large banana)
- Blueberries and blackberries (¾ cup)
- Grapefruit (½)
- Grapes (4 ounces or ⅔ cup, 15–17 grapes)
- Kiwi (4 ounces)
- Mango (⅔ cup slices)
- Nectarine (4 ounces)
- Pear (4 ounces)
- Pineapple (4 ounces or ¾ cup chunks)
- Plum (4 ounces)
- Raspberries (1 cup)
- Strawberries (1¼ cup)

- Cantaloupe (¼ of a 20-ounce melon or 1 cup pieces)
- Cherries (12 cherries)
- Fruit salad (½ cup)
- Orange (7 ounces with skin)
- Peach (8 ounces)
- Watermelon (1¼ cup cubes or 10-ounce slice with skin)
- Tangerine (4 ounces)

100-Calorie Snack List

1. ⅛ cup or 2 tablespoons any nut (no-carb choice)
2. 2 ak-mak® crackers (6 g carb) or 2 Wasa Crisp'n Light® crackers (7 g carb) or 1 Joseph's® whole wheat/oat bran pita (4 g carb) and 1 slice 2% milk cheese or 1 light string cheese
3. ⅛ cup pineapple with ½ cup low-fat cottage cheese (8 g carb)
4. 6 stalks celery with either 2 teaspoons peanut butter or 2 Laughing Cow® light wedges (no-carb choice)
5. 6 ounces light yogurt or 6 ounces Greek plain yogurt sweetened with Splenda® or Equal® (read yogurt nutrition labels for carb grams)
6. 1 fruit serving (15 g carb) or 6 ounces skim or 1% milk (12 g carb) and 1 tablespoon nuts
7. 100-calorie Balance Bar® (see nutrition labels for carb grams)
8. 2 tablespoons hummus and 6 stalks celery or 12 carrots (15 g carb)

200-Calorie Snack List

1. ¼ cup any nut (no-carb choice)
2. ⅓ cup pineapple with 1 cup low-fat cottage cheese (18 g carb)
3. 8 celery stalks with 1½ tablespoons peanut butter (no-carb choice)
4. 6 ounces light yogurt or 8 ounces skim or 1% milk and 2 tablespoons nuts (12 g carb)
5. 4 ak-mak® (12 g carb) or 4 Wasa Crisp'n Light® crackers (14 g carb) and 2 light string cheeses or 2 slices 2% milk cheese or 1 tablespoon peanut butter
6. 1 fruit serving (15 g carb) with 1½ tablespoons peanut butter

7. 2 eggs poached, hard-boiled or scrambled in 1 tablespoon skim milk and 1 small whole wheat pita (4 g carb) or 1 slice low-carb/light whole wheat bread (7 g carb)

8. 210-calorie Zone® bar or Balance Bar® (see nutrition label for carb grams)

9. Fiber One® or Kashi® bar or Nature Valley® chewy bar and 1 tablespoon nuts (see nutrition label for carb grams)

10. 100-calorie snack from 100-calorie snack list and 2 tablespoons nuts (15 g carb)

11. 4 celery stalks and 2 tablespoons walnuts and 2 tablespoons light cream cheese (no-carb choice)

12. 100-calorie bag microwave popcorn (5 cups popped) and 2 tablespoons nuts (15 g carb)

Meal Plan Tricks of the Trade

1. At lunch feel free to have salad, raw vegetables or cooked vegetables. You can then add the fat serving in with the salad or vegetables. If you want to add cheese or nuts to the salad, you must then use balsamic or white wine vinegar or lemon juice as your dressing choice to avoid adding extra calories. Some other ideas are melting cheese on frozen veggies, adding peanut butter to celery or dipping cut up veggies into light dressing. Beware that fat-free dressings add carbohydrates and should not be used.

2. There are some drinks you can have in unlimited quantities. These include flavored waters such as Propel Zero®, Fruit 2O®, Aquafina® and Dasani®, Crystal Light®, seltzers, diet soda, coffee, tea, other diet drinks like Diet V8 Splash® or Diet Snapple® and, of course, water. Caffeine can interfere with how well your insulin works, though, so try to keep a lid on how much of it you take in through beverages like coffee, tea, caffeinated waters and diet sodas.

3. If you are hungry and want to eat beyond the plan, you can always have more vegetables or salad. You can also make a broth-based vegetable soup, but be sure to use low-sodium, fat-free chicken broth as a base.

4. You can have sugar-free Jell-O® with a dollop of light or fat-free Cool Whip® if you really feel you need something sweet, but don't eat more than four servings per day. Other sugar-free products are also options, but make sure to check the calorie content as sugar-free doesn't necessarily mean calorie-free.

5. It will help if you purchase measuring cups and a food scale to assist you with portion control with the menus.

6. Acceptable trans fat-free spreads are as follows: Smart Balance®, Promise Heart Health Essentials®, Olivio®, I Can't Believe It's Not Butter! Light® and Brummel & Brown®. You may also use butter spray, Molly McButter®, Butter Buds® or olive oil in a spray can.

7. You are free to use artificial sweeteners, including Splenda®, Equal® and Sweet'N Low®.

8. If you cannot finish both Lean Cuisine®, Healthy Choice® or Smart Ones® dinners and you choose to eat only one, you can add another 200-calorie snack at some other time of day as needed.

9. Seasonings and spices are unlimited.

10. For the snacks, any type of peanut butter can be used, but natural peanut butter is preferable. Also, any type of unsalted nut is acceptable.

11. Olive and canola oils are the preferred oils for cooking and use on salads.

12. You can use fat-free half-and-half or milk in coffee, both of which are preferable to using cream.

SET UP A MEAL PLAN LOGBOOK

In order to learn what approaches to take for your specific long-term weight and blood glucose control strategies, you'll need to learn first what your current patterns are when it comes to eating, exercising and controlling your diabetes. Your logbook is a great tool to help you become a detective, so to speak, in investigating your patterns of behavior. Its purpose is to make you more aware and conscious of your behaviors and help you learn from your patterns since you must first recognize an unproductive behavior before you can change it.

Make copies of the daily menu plan logbook that follows, keep them in your notebook and fill out each day on the plan. You'll notice that you have to check your blood glucose frequently, rate your feelings of hunger, choose snacks from lists provided and use a meal replacement for breakfast and lunch—at least initially. You can choose to substitute healthy foods in place of meal replacement shakes, but we suggest that you give them a try for at least the first six weeks to really kick-start your weight loss and then wean yourself off of them gradually. As mentioned, daily menu ideas can be found in the appendices.

DAILY MENU PLAN LOGBOOK DATE:	CHECK ✔	TIME:	HUNGER LEVEL: Choose 1–5*	NOTES/COMMENTS:
BREAKFAST **BLOOD GLUCOSE**				
Meal Replacement				
LUNCH **BLOOD GLUCOSE**				
Meal Replacement				
Vegetable Serving/ Salad				
1-2 Fat Servings (1 for 1500, 2 for 1800)				
Fruit Serving (1800)				

DINNER **BLOOD GLUCOSE**			
Menu Selection Number			
Snack #1			
Snack #2			
Snack #3 (if applicable)			
BEDTIME **BLOOD GLUCOSE**			

* 1 is defined as starving and 5 is defined as stuffed.
Adapted from Joslin Diabetes Center Why WAIT program materials. Copyright © 2012 by Joslin Diabetes Center (www.joslin.org). All rights reserved.

UNDERSTAND METABOLISM, PHYSICAL ACTIVITY AND EXERCISE

Let's spend a few minutes now defining some of the terms that we'll be using, starting with *metabolism*. What does this term actually mean? In short, metabolism is the process of converting food to energy, but it also refers to the speed with which your body burns calories. Your metabolism is influenced by your age (naturally slowing down by about 5 percent per decade after age 40); sex (men generally burn more calories at rest than women); and proportion of lean body mass (the more muscle you have, the higher your metabolic rate is).

It's also important to distinguish between exercise and physical activity since, although they are often used interchangeably, they actually mean different things. Physical activity uses your muscles, but doesn't necessarily elevate your heart rate or increase breathing very much. Some examples of common physical activities include easy walking, vacuuming, mowing the lawn and doing laundry.

Exercise is a specific type of physical activity that is more structured and intentional, with the purpose of improving your endurance and strength. It is repetitive, uses big muscle groups and elevates your heart rate. The reason this distinction is important is that you may get plenty of physical activity going about your daily activities, but you may not get enough exercise to reap all of the benefits. Examples of exercise include going for a brisk walk, biking, swimming and training with resistance bands.

EXERCISE USES GLUCOSE AND FAT

Glucose, the body's main form of energy during exercise, can be found in the bloodstream, muscles and liver. As you know, any carbohydrate food is ultimately converted to glucose. Some of it gets used right away, but more is usually stored in the liver and muscles. During the first few minutes of exercise, your muscles utilize the glucose stored in the muscles almost exclusively. As you exercise, your body releases stress hormones, adrenaline and other hormones that signal to your liver that your body needs more glucose and your liver responds by producing and releasing the needed glucose into the bloodstream.

After approximately 20 minutes of exercise, your body begins to use slightly more stored fat for energy. Body fat is an internal energy source since the fat that we eat is not used immediately and gets stored for later use. Its use is also dependent on things like how hard you're working (more intense exercise uses more glucose and stored carbohydrates), how long you exercise (longer duration requires greater fat contributions) and how frequently you exercise (as it takes a while to fully restore your carbohydrates in your muscles and liver).

What you need to remember is that you're always burning calories during exercise and it doesn't really matter whether they come from glucose or fat because the more calories you burn (from either source), the more weight loss you can expect. You need to burn around 3500 calories to lose one pound of fat. To lose weight, however, you need to exercise every day and combining this activity with cutting back calories every day from your meal plan will help you reach your weight loss target.

Calorie reduction and exercise are the two components we focus on most in the Diabetes Breakthrough program. For example, if you cut back 600 calories a day from your meal plan and burn 400 calories with exercise, you may lose about two pounds per week.

BENEFITS FROM EXERCISE AND PHYSICAL ACTIVITY

Do you know what all the many benefits of being physically active are? Becoming more active obviously helps with weight control, which is why it's such an integral part of this program. In addition, exercise improves your blood glucose, blood pressure and cholesterol. It can even make you feel happier and give you more energy.

Equally important is the fact that exercise increases the effectiveness of your medications by making your insulin work better. Taking a lot of medications can be expensive, so cost can be a motivator for you to exercise because it should reduce the amount of medications you need to take. Given all of these great benefits of exercise, you really need to start thinking about exercise as your new medication. Later on in this book, we'll also talk in more detail about how resistance exercise builds muscle strength and increases metabolism.

Benefits of Exercise/Physical Activity

- Helps you lose weight and keep it off.
- Reduces how much belly fat you have.
- Improves blood glucose control and A1C.
- Makes you feel better.
- Helps medications work better.
- Increases your metabolism.
- Helps lower resting blood pressure.
- Raises good cholesterol (HDL) levels.
- Increases your muscle strength.
- Improves the function of your blood vessels.
- Improves your posture.
- Improves state of mind.

WHICH TYPES OF EXERCISE SHOULD YOU DO?

Aerobic exercise: Also known as cardiovascular or "cardio" exercise, this type of physical activity works your muscles, heart and cardiovascular system. The heart is a muscle and aerobic exercise strengthens it, but when you want to get it stronger, you have to work it just like any other muscle. Diabetes and the risk for heart disease come as a package and it is our goal to protect you from any heart problems, so we will be guiding you in increasing your daily aerobic exercise as you make progress through the Diabetes Breakthrough program.

Resistance training: Whether it's called resistance, strength or weight training, during this activity your muscles work against a force (weights, bands) or gravity, which helps to strengthen them. For this program, you don't need to join a gym (unless you want to) since you can easily start with some hand weights (or household items) and resistance bands and slowly increase the amount of weight or the resistance of the bands.

Flexibility exercise: Muscles contract repeatedly with exercise and may be overworked to a certain extent, the result being that they can get stiff or sore afterward. It is important to perform static stretching exercises to allow loosening your muscles in order to improve flexibility and the range of motion at your joints, which can also help prevent injury. The best time to stretch is when your muscles are warm. Keep in mind that stretching is separate from warming up and cooling down for your aerobic exercise.

DON'T FORGET TO WARM UP AND COOL DOWN

The warm-up is some easier exercise that comes before your aerobic or resistance workout to increase blood flow and put oxygen into your muscles. For instance, if walking is your chosen form of exercise, to warm up, you could walk at a slow speed for two to five minutes, or if you're doing resistance training, you can warm up by doing a movement with little or no resistance to start. The aerobic ("conditioning") phase follows the warm-up and may consist of an activity at a faster pace like walking at moderate intensity for 30 to 40 minutes. The cooldown is the last phase of your activity during which you slowly reduce your heart rate by walking at a slower pace for another three to five minutes before stopping.

The warm-up and cooldown portions do not count as part of your target workout time since they are done at a much lower intensity than your conditioning phase. Stretching usually follows the cooldown, but can also be done after your warm-up or any time that your muscles or joints start to feel tight during an activity.

GET STARTED BEING MORE ACTIVE

The main focus of the exercise program is to increase your muscle mass and strength and to challenge the muscles to burn more calories. In addition, you will learn advanced types of training that will make your exercise routine more efficient. Your exercise plan progresses over the 12 weeks of this program. This week, you'll start by doing 20 minutes of an aerobic exercise for four days. Over the course of 12 weeks, you will gradually work up to doing 50 to 60 minutes of exercise six days a week.

If it's hard for you to do all 20 minutes at one time initially, you can split your sessions into two shorter bouts of 10 minutes each. Splitting up workouts into several shorter bouts throughout the day can aid in reaching the recommended target for how long you should exercise each day. Just be sure that you do at least 10 minutes per bout, if possible.

While any activity that uses your large muscle groups in a rhythmic way over a period of two minutes or more is considered aerobic, feel free to pick the activities that best suit you. Some examples of aerobic activities that you can perform for 20 minutes for four days this week include walking, jogging/running, cycling, rowing, swimming, arm biking, aerobic exercise classes, aerobic machines such as the elliptical trainer, recumbent bike or cross trainer, conditioning machines, free weights, resistance bands, Zumba and other forms of dancing.

You will be learning how to do circuit, interval, superset and core training as we go along and you'll have plenty of practice each week. We're going to work on all of these components in order to improve your exercise plan, help you lose weight and better manage your diabetes.

YOUR EXERCISE PLAN FOR WEEK 1

This week you'll just be getting started with some easy aerobic activity. Stretching is also important to do when you're active and will be covered this week (and included every week from here on out).

WEEK 1: DIABETES BREAKTHROUGH EXERCISE PLAN

DAY	AEROBIC	RESISTANCE	STRETCHING	TYPES OF EXERCISE
1	17 minutes		3 minutes	Aerobic
2	17 minutes		3 minutes	Stretching
3				
4	17 minutes		3 minutes	
5	17 minutes		3 minutes	
6				
7				

TOTAL TIME: 20 MINUTES

HOW HARD SHOULD YOU WORK OUT?

How do you know how hard to exercise? A good way to determine whether you should speed up or slow down is by using the "talk test." Exercising at a moderate intensity—meaning that you can still manage to carry on a conversation during your activity—is optimal because it indicates that you are working hard enough to strengthen your heart muscle but not so hard that you can't sustain the activity long enough to gain its benefits. If you can sing or whistle while doing the activity, the speed or intensity is too low and you likely need to speed up. If you're short of breath or winded and can't talk, you are exercising vigorously and may need to slow down (especially when you're just starting out).

There are a few other methods of determining intensity, as well. One is using a measure of overall perceived exertion, which is how hard you feel you are working based on sensations you are having related to your increased heart and breathing rates, increased sweating and muscle fatigue. Although this is a subjective measure, your exertion rating provides a fairly good estimate of your actual heart rate during physical activity. A rating of "somewhat hard" to "hard" suggests that physical activity is being performed at a moderate level.

At any point, if you have joint, muscle or chest pain, you should stop and possibly check with your health care provider if the pain doesn't subside immediately or recurs every time you exercise. In that case, you may need to explore some other, less painful options for your exercise.

WHEN SHOULD YOU WORK OUT?

We always say that the best time to exercise is when you can make the time during the day. There is no one particular time of day that is best for exercise, so stick with your personal preferences. However, if you exercise in the evening, one benefit is that when you wake up, your fasting blood glucose may be lower because exercise keeps the glucose "doors" open for 24 to 48 hours, as we talked about earlier. For anyone on insulin, however, you may need to reduce your rapid-acting insulin doses by one to two units at dinner if you plan to exercise later in the evening, to avoid nocturnal hypoglycemia (low blood glucose during the night). If your doses are too high, insulin may make your blood glucose level too low. If you feel shaky, sweaty or confused (i.e., symptoms of low blood glucose), check your glucose and take 15 grams of glucose or another sugar (such as regular soda or hard candy) if it's below 70 mg/dl.

Keep in mind that early morning exercise done before eating anything can cause a rise in your blood glucose levels instead. To prevent this from occurring, eat a small snack before you exercise to make your body release a little bit of insulin. Just a small amount of food and insulin breaks your overnight fast and lowers your level of insulin resistance, which is generally highest in the morning before breakfast.

Essential Components of Your Weekly Planned Exercise
- Aerobic exercise.
- Resistance exercise.
- Stretching exercise.
- Extra daily movement (unplanned).

LEARN FROM YOUR ACTIVITY LOGBOOK

You can use the following as your primary daily exercise logbook. Added together with your SMART goals, dietary log, daily step goals and resistance training log that you'll be starting in Week 4, you have the potential to learn a lot from your comprehensive logbook.

DATE/ TIME	BLOOD GLUCOSE BEFORE	TYPE OF EXERCISE	BLOOD GLUCOSE AFTER	MINUTES OF EXERCISE
		Walking outside or on treadmill		
		Biking		
		Conditioning machine		
		Swimming or other water exercise		
		Other:		
		Resistance exercise		
		Stretching	Check ☐	

Notes/Comments:

WHY STRETCHING IS GOOD FOR YOU

Let's talk more about stretching, which should be incorporated into every exercise session. Stretching has many benefits performed either on its own or along with aerobic and/or resistance training. It helps prevent stiffness after your workout and helps you accomplish your daily activities more easily by increasing the range of motion you have in your joints.

Blood glucose levels, when poorly controlled, cause you to lose flexibility faster than normal aging alone does—which is all the more reason to not only stretch frequently, but also control your blood glucose levels more effectively. Inflexible joints lead to greater rates of injuries, as well as limited movement and a lesser ability to balance and stay on your feet at all times.

Benefits of Stretching
- Helps avoid stiff, sore and tired muscles.
- Helps you move and reach.
- Helps avoid injuries.
- Combats the loss of flexibility caused by aging, disuse and diabetes.

HOW TO STRETCH

It's important to remember to stretch after you've warmed up, not before. When your muscles are cold, they're like a cold piece of taffy: not very pliable and more prone to injury. A warmed muscle is less likely to be pulled or injured because it's more flexible. The best time to stretch is at the end of your workout when your muscles are at their warmest. Of course, you can stretch at the beginning of exercise or any time during it, but be sure you warm up at least a little first. Some people benefit from doing gentle stretches after their initial warm-up and then deeper stretches at the end of the workout. Experiment and see what works best for you.

To stretch safely, find the position where you can feel the stretch, but not any pain and hold that position for at least 20 to 30 seconds and repeat each stretch twice. You should never bounce when stretching—rather, just hold your muscle in its lengthened position and relax. It's also okay to do dynamic stretching, which involves slow, gentle movement to induce the stretch, but not bouncing movements. Stretching should never be painful. If it is, decrease the stretch or change position to relieve the pain. We're all built differently, so not every stretch is right for everyone.

Principles of Effective Stretching

- Perform stretching exercises when muscles are warm.
- Perform stretching exercises in a slow, controlled manner.
- Do a static stretching routine, or do dynamic stretching that involves slow movement.
- Hold a static stretch for 15 to 60 seconds and repeat each stretch twice.
- Stretch to a point of tightness, without inducing discomfort.
- Never do a bouncing movement when stretching or you may injure yourself.

EASY STRETCHING EXERCISES

For all of these stretches, it is recommended that you hold them for about 15 to 60 seconds, at the point that you can feel the stretch but no discomfort and ideally repeat each stretch twice.

1. **NECK—Neck Stretch**

   While tilting head to the left, pull right arm down with left hand until stretch is felt. Hold for about 15 seconds and repeat on other side of neck.

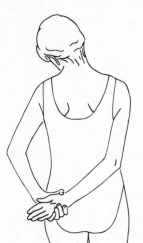

2. **SHOULDERS—Posterior Deltoids/ Rhomboids Stretch**

   Pull arm across chest until stretch is felt. Turn head away from pull and hold. Repeat with other arm.

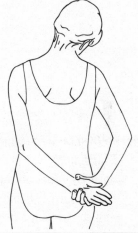
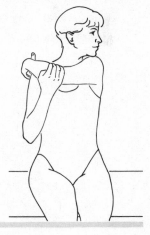

3. SHOULDERS—Extensors Stretch

With hands on wall or rail and feet shoulder-width apart, move chest forward toward floor. Hold stretch and repeat.

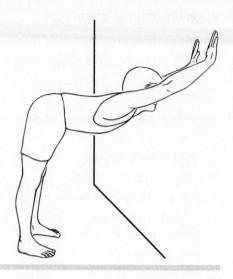

4. HIP/KNEE—Hamstring Stretch (Standing)

Place right foot on stool. Slowly lean forward, keeping back straight, until stretch is felt in back of thigh. Hold and then repeat with other leg. For an additional stretch, place leg up on a taller object to increase range of motion.

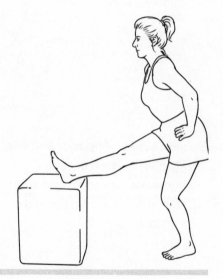

5. HIP/KNEE—Hip Flexor Stretch

With right leg supported by holding onto
a bar or chair, slowly bend the other leg
until stretch is felt in the thigh of the bent
leg. Hold stretch and repeat
with other leg.

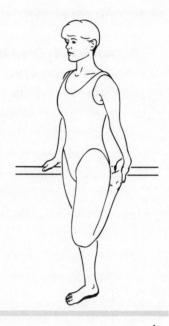

6. LOWER LEG—Calf Stretch

Keeping back leg straight, with
heel on floor and slightly turned
outward, lean into wall until
a stretch is felt in calf of the
straight leg. Hold and repeat with
other leg.

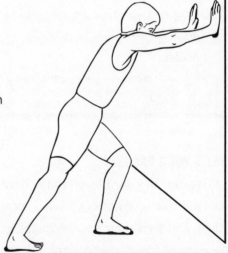

Physical Activity Checklist for Safety

- Follow the exercise plan discussed in this chapter and progress, as you are able, to doing 60 minutes, 6 days per week (as listed in the 12-week exercise progression plan).
- Wear comfortable clothes, socks and shoes.
- Always have your blood glucose meter and snacks with you (e.g., glucose tablets, regular soda, hard candy, juice or other snacks either to prevent or treat low blood glucose).
- Check your blood glucose before exercise to learn your body's unique response.
- Blood glucose goals before exercise:
  - Diabetes pills and/or Byetta, Bydureon or Victoza: over 90 mg/dl
  - Insulin only: over 110 mg/dl
  - Insulin plus diabetes pills, or insulin plus Symlin: over 110 mg/dl
- Take 15 grams of carbohydrates if your blood glucose is below your goal.
- Keep records of exercise/physical activity in your daily/weekly logbook.
- Wear or carry medical identification, especially when exercising outdoors.
- Drink water during physical activity to stay adequately hydrated.

WHAT'S YOUR EXCUSE?

At this point in your life, you may have lost weight on diets and gained it back (and often even more), started exercise programs and then dropped out of them and seen some improvements in your blood glucose levels that may have relapsed into poorer control. The problem with making plans and setting goals—even SMART ones—is that things don't always work out the way you expect them to. Nevertheless, you will likely have some ideas about what has presented you with a particular challenge (or trigger for a slip) in your past.

This week, you're going to brainstorm about what you'll do when barriers come up and get in the way of your goals. You can start by identifying patterns that emerge both when things are going as planned and when they are feeling more challenging—and the way to go about doing this is by using a logbook to record when you accomplish or don't reach your planned goals.

WHAT KEEPS YOU FROM BEING MORE ACTIVE?

A good first step in staying on track is to pinpoint what's getting in your way. This week, take the quiz to see which areas you need to focus on to get and keep yourself moving in the right direction. Then set SMART goals to try to overcome these barriers this week.

Barriers to Being Active Quiz

Directions: Listed below are reasons that people give to describe why they do not get as much physical activity as they think they should. Please read each statement and indicate how likely you are to say each of the following statements (Very likely = completely agree; Very unlikely = completely disagree):

HOW LIKELY ARE YOU TO SAY?	VERY LIKELY	SOMEWHAT LIKELY	SOMEWHAT UNLIKELY	VERY UNLIKELY
1. My day is so busy now; I just don't think I can make the time to include physical activity in my regular schedule.	3	2	1	0
2. None of my family members or friends like to do anything active, so I don't have a chance to exercise.	3	2	1	0
3. I'm just too tired after work to get any exercise.	3	2	1	0
4. I've been thinking about getting more exercise, but I just can't seem to get started.	3	2	1	0
5. I'm getting older so exercise can be risky.	3	2	1	0

continued

HOW LIKELY ARE YOU TO SAY?	VERY LIKELY	SOMEWHAT LIKELY	SOMEWHAT UNLIKELY	VERY UNLIKELY
6. I don't get enough exercise because I have never learned the skills for any sport.	3	2	1	0
7. I don't have access to jogging trails, swimming pools, bike paths, etc.	3	2	1	0
8. Physical activity takes too much time away from other commitments—time, work, family, etc.	3	2	1	0
9. I'm embarrassed about how I will look when I exercise with others.	3	2	1	0
10. I don't get enough sleep as it is. I just couldn't get up early or stay up late to get some exercise.	3	2	1	0
11. It's easier for me to find excuses not to exercise than to go out to do something.	3	2	1	0
12. I know of too many people who have hurt themselves by overdoing it with exercise.	3	2	1	0
13. I really can't see learning a new sport at my age.	3	2	1	0
14. It's just too expensive. You have to take a class or join a club or buy the right equipment.	3	2	1	0
15. My free times during the day are too short to include exercise.	3	2	1	0

16. My usual social activities with family or friends do not include physical activity.	3	2	1	0
17. I'm too tired during the week and I need the weekend to catch up on my rest.	3	2	1	0
18. I want to get more exercise, but I just can't seem to make myself stick to anything.	3	2	1	0
19. I'm afraid I might injure myself or have a heart attack.	3	2	1	0
20. I'm not good enough at any physical activity to make it fun.	3	2	1	0
21. If we had exercise facilities and showers at work, then I would be more likely to exercise.	3	2	1	0

Available online at http://www.cdc.gov/nccdphp/dnpa/physical/life/barriers_quiz.pdf

Follow these instructions to score yourself:

- Enter the circled number in the spaces provided in the following score chart, putting together the number for statement 1 on line 1, statement 2 on line 2 and so on.
- Add the three scores on each line. Your barriers to physical activity fall into one or more of seven categories: lack of time, social influences, lack of energy, lack of willpower, fear of injury, lack of skill and lack of resources.
- A score of five or above in any category shows that this is an important barrier for you to overcome.

____ + ____ + ____ = _____
1   8   15   Lack of time

____ + ____ + ____ = _____
2   9   16   Social influences

____ + ____ + ____ = _____
3   10   17   Lack of energy

____ + ____ + ____ = _____
4   11   18   Lack of willpower

____ + ____ + ____ = _____
5   12   19   Fear of injury

____ + ____ + ____ = _____
6   13   20   Lack of skill

____ + ____ + ____ = _____
7   14   21   Lack of resources

FOLLOW THE ABCs OF BEHAVIOR CHANGE

When you look at everything you put into your logbook each week, think about the ABCs of behavior change. This approach of using the ABCs is a great way to train yourself to notice the behavior patterns that you want to change.

A stands for **activating event.** This is the trigger for the behavior; for example, eating at a certain restaurant that serves rolls that you really love before your meal arrives may lead you to eat them.

B is the **behavior** pattern that the trigger sets off. In this case, maybe the pattern is that you eat two or three rolls before your meal arrives without even realizing it because you're busy talking and they taste so good.

C are the **consequences** of the behavior, or what results from it. Using the same example, the consequence may be that you eat way more carbohydrates or calories than is healthy for you and you feel really bad about it.

TRIGGERS CAN LEAD YOU DOWN THE WRONG PATH

Let's look specifically at triggers, which often fall into certain patterns related to timing, types of food, activities or situations and feelings. For instance, certain times of day, days during the week or seasons may cause you to have a harder time sticking to a health plan. Or it may be certain types of food that are hard for you to manage in a portion-controlled way. For others of you, it may be certain activities, situations or special events (e.g., holidays, parties, watching TV, work-related meetings or vacations) that are harder for you to manage. We are not asking you to completely give up those activities, but you'll need to come up with ways to keep your eating, exercise and diabetes on track while still enjoying the event. Some of you may find that you have certain feelings that are triggers for you to slip away from healthier behaviors, such as boredom, loneliness, anger, sadness, stress and even celebration. Here, too, it will be important to learn new ways of managing these potentially triggering emotions differently.

Can you think of a trigger in any of these categories and effective ways that you have handled it in the past? This week, start using your logbook to identify your unique triggers, challenges and barriers to ongoing weight loss. Each week, you'll also start to identify these triggers and creatively come up with solutions to overcome many barriers ahead of time.

By looking at your weekly logbook, you will start to notice certain patterns that seem unique about your eating and exercise habits. You'll then be able to better recognize potential patterns for when you are likely to be tempted to eat or fall off your exercise plan. Changing your response to these triggers may help you stick to a healthier plan.

IDENTIFY YOUR TRIGGERS

Think about your unique triggers and write down as many of them as come to mind. Next week, check to see how many of these same triggers show up in your logbook.

A: Activating event—What is triggering the behavior?

B: Behavior—Describe the behavior pattern.

C: Consequences—What results from the behavior? How do you feel afterward?

TIMING: WHEN DO YOU EAT ACCORDING TO YOUR PLAN AND WHEN ARE YOU MOST LIKELY TO GO OFF TRACK? (THINK SEASONALLY, TIME OF DAY, TIMING IN THE WEEK)

_____

_____

_____

_____

TYPES OF FOOD: WHAT TYPES OF FOODS CAN YOU MANAGE PORTION SIZE WELL AND WHAT FOODS ARE TRIGGERS TO OVERDO IT? (HIGH-RISK FOODS)

_____

_____

_____

_____

ACTIVITY OR SITUATION: WHAT SORTS OF SITUATIONS OR ACTIVITIES HAVE BECOME CONNECTED TO THE HABIT OF OVEREATING? (WATCHING TV, MEETINGS AT WORK, ETC.)

_____

_____

_____

_____

FEELINGS: WHAT FEELINGS ARE TYPICAL TRIGGERS FOR OVEREATING? BOREDOM, LONELINESS, ANGER, SADNESS, ANXIETY OR CELEBRATIONS?

_____

_____

_____

_____

HAPPILY PRAYING ON HER KNEES AGAIN

Remember Donna, who said that she prayed for the guidance that led her to this program? She recalls, "The first time I went to the program I had to use a recumbent bike that didn't hurt my knees." Now two years later, she has lost a total of 100 pounds and she no longer is in the "diabetes" range with her overall blood glucose readings, plus she's off all of her medications. She's still exercising, managing her food intake and losing weight, slowly and steadily.

Even more exciting to her, though, is seeing her progress in real-life terms. Although her arthritic pain in her knees kept her off of them at the start of the program, she happily recounts, "Recently, I was able to get down on my knees to pray with my grandkids for the first time in a very long time. You'll never know how much this program changed my life."

DIABETES BREAKTHROUGH WEEK 2

*Medications and Weight Gain, Diabetes Pills,
Serving Sizes and Cross Training*

The weight you have gained over time is likely one of the contributing factors to your development of type 2 diabetes or prediabetes, but many people with type 1 diabetes also develop symptoms and consequences of insulin resistance when they gain weight. Losing weight can be an issue for anyone with either type of diabetes because of the balancing act required among diet, medications, exercise, stress and other factors that can impact insulin needs.

This week, you'll continue with the meal plan you started last week and advance a little with your physical activity. You'll practice balancing out what you're eating with what you're doing to burn more calories and you'll get some help tackling your problem eating. What's more, you will begin to learn more about the effects of your medications on weight gain and ways you may be able to adjust your meds to help yourself lose more weight on this program.

WEIGHT GAIN IS NOT JUST FOR TYPE 2 DIABETES

As a 58-year-old male with type 1 diabetes for most of his life, David was horrified when he calculated his body mass index (BMI) and found that it was above 30, putting him squarely in the "obese" category. And he's not alone since the latest projections estimate that half of American adults will be classified as obese by 2030—less than two decades from now.

"I'd never thought of myself as being obese before, even though I'd been gaining weight slowly over the years," David says. "But when I saw my weight, I decided that I needed to do something about it." A recent Joslin 50-year medalist (meaning that he was recognized for being on insulin for five decades), he'd seen what diabetes can do to others when it's not well controlled. David has kept his blood glucose levels in check, but found that he needed more and more insulin due to becoming resistant to insulin. Unfortunately for him, taking more insulin to maintain control over his blood glucose also predisposed him to gaining more weight—a vicious cycle that makes weight management extremely difficult. You'll hear more of his story about his weight loss later in this chapter.

LOSE THE MEDICATIONS TO LOSE THE WEIGHT (AND VICE VERSA)

Despite what diet books and reality TV shows may want you to believe, losing weight—especially when you have diabetes—is not just about deprivation, hard work and self-control. We're here to let you know how some of your diabetes medications may have been conspiring against you to keep you heavier, despite your valiant attempts to lose weight, and what you can do about it. Our focus on the effects of medications on weight loss and how losing weight also affects your medication needs is one component that makes this program truly unique.

What do you really know about your medications? Did you know that some of them usually cause weight gain? More important, did you know that many of them can actually help you lose weight if you use them in place of other ones? Your doctor may not be as up-to-date on how many of the newer medications affect your body weight. But you'll soon know a lot more about how they work, which ones are weight-friendly and which ones cause weight gain, making you a lot more prepared to discuss with your doctor or other health care provider how to reduce or modify them when you start losing weight.

TAKE THIS VERY SHORT MEDICATIONS QUIZ TO FIND OUT HOW MUCH
YOU ALREADY KNOW (OR DON'T KNOW):

1. All of the following diabetes medications are weight-friendly,
    meaning that they can help you lose weight or won't cause
    weight gain, EXCEPT for

    a. Metformin (Glucophage)

    b. Insulin

    c. Januvia, Onglyza, Tradjenta, Nesina and Galvus

    d. Byetta and Bydureon

    e. Victoza

    f. Invokana

2. All of the following diabetes medications cause weight gain,
    EXCEPT for

    a. Insulin

    b. Actos, Avandia

    c. Sulfonylureas (e.g., glyburide, glipizide, glimepiride)

    d. Glinides (i.e., Starlix, Prandin)

    e. Victoza

P.S. The answers are: (1) b (insulin) and (2) e (Victoza).

UNDERSTAND HOW YOUR MEDICATIONS WORK

In addition to carbohydrates that you eat, your liver, pancreas, stomach,
kidneys and muscles play a role in regulating your blood glucose levels. As
we've discussed, glucose comes from the breakdown of carbohydrate foods
that we eat. Food is digested in your gastrointestinal system, which allows
glucose to enter the bloodstream. You need insulin to help your body use this
glucose effectively for energy. Insulin also stimulates the body to store glucose
as glycogen. The liver contains the most significant and most accessible store
of glycogen that can be used to manage blood glucose levels when blood glucose is low. Think of the liver as your bank: you save your extra cash in it and
you withdraw that money when you need it. Muscles also store glycogen, but
that's for their own use during exercise and can't be used to raise your blood

glucose levels. Kidneys filter glucose and reabsorb it back to the blood. If this mechanism is blocked, glucose appears in excess in the urine and becomes lower in the blood. Finally, the pancreas is very important because along with producing insulin, it also produces glucagon, the hormone that tells the liver to release glucose from its glycogen stores (like withdrawing money from the bank). Each of these organs can have a large impact on blood glucose.

Your medications actually target one or more of these organs to control your blood glucose levels. There are many choices for oral and injectable medications including insulin and they all work differently. Knowing how your medications work and their potential side effects is important, particularly since you now know that some diabetes medications cause you to gain weight while others help you lose it.

With the knowledge you gain from this book, you'll be ready and able to approach your own health care provider about helping you select the best weight-friendly medication(s) for you. As you lose weight, your health care team will likely also have to adjust your medications in order to maximize their benefit without causing problems with low blood glucose levels.

Diabetes Pills and Injectables

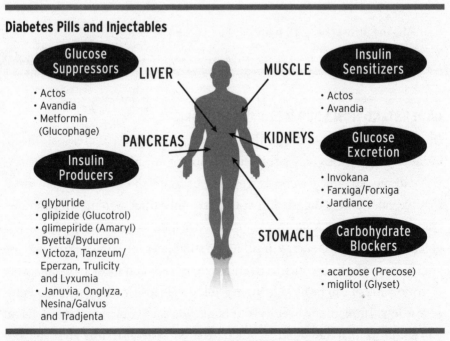

Glucose Suppressors   **LIVER**
- Actos
- Avandia
- Metformin (Glucophage)

MUSCLE   **Insulin Sensitizers**
- Actos
- Avandia

PANCREAS

KIDNEYS   **Glucose Excretion**
- Invokana
- Farxiga/Forxiga
- Jardiance

Insulin Producers
- glyburide
- glipizide (Glucotrol)
- glimepiride (Amaryl)
- Byetta/Bydureon
- Victoza, Tanzeum/Eperzan, Trulicity and Lyxumia
- Januvia, Onglyza, Nesina/Galvus and Tradjenta

STOMACH   **Carbohydrate Blockers**
- acarbose (Precose)
- miglitol (Glyset)

Know Your Medications

What should you know about your medications? Minimally, you should know the following:

- Name (brand name and generic name, if available) and type of medication.
- How it works and when to take it.
- What to do if you miss a dose.
- What to watch for (potential side effects).

You really need to know the names of your medications and not just be able to identify different ones as "the green pill" or "the blue pill." If you are taking many medications (for diabetes and other health conditions) or have trouble remembering information about them, write the information down and keep it in your wallet. Remember to update your list of medications whenever you make a change.

When it comes to your medications, you should additionally know their brand names and their generic names (in case one is available at a lower price) and the correct dosage, as well as when to take your medication in relation to food intake to ensure that it's working most effectively. For example, metformin (brand name Glucophage) and Actos need to be taken with a meal. To work most effectively, sulfonylureas, such as glyburide (sold as multiple brand names), Glucotrol (generic glipizide) and Amaryl (generic glimepiride), should be taken before a meal, while carbohydrate blockers like Precose (acarbose) or Glyset (miglitol) are taken along with your first bite. Newer medications including Januvia, Onglyza, Tradjenta, Nesina, Galvus, Invokana, Farxiga (U.S.A.), Forxiga (Europe) and Jardiance can be taken before or after your meal.

If you miss a scheduled dosage of your medication, don't take an extra dose. Just take your next dose at its scheduled time and be sure to record the missed dose in your logbook. If you miss a dose of insulin, however, you should check with your health care provider about whether you need to try to replace any of the dosage or take a different type of insulin to cover the loss over the short run.

WHAT IS A "WEIGHT-FRIENDLY" MEDICATION?

Tight blood glucose control often comes at a price: increased weight gain and more frequent hypoglycemia. From a body-weight perspective, medications that lower blood glucose levels are classified into two groups: those known to promote weight gain ("weight fury" medications) and those that are weight neutral (causing neither loss nor gain) or associated with weight loss or minimal weight gain ("weight-friendly" ones). The more you know about which category your medications fall in, the easier you can work with your health care team to adjust your medications to make your weight loss easier.

We know that this approach works because we've already proven that it does. Most Why WAIT program participants have been able to cut their diabetes medications by 50 to 60 percent after losing weight and many of them have stopped taking them altogether and no longer have diabetes. In fact, 21 percent on short-acting insulin are off of it in just 12 weeks. For others, their daily doses of long- and/or short-acting insulin have been cut back by around 55 percent.

PICK WEIGHT-FRIENDLY MEDICATIONS TO LOSE WEIGHT

A central part of the Joslin Why WAIT program is our focus on reducing diabetes medications that contribute to weight gain and replacing them (if needed) with ones that are weight-friendly because they don't affect body weight, they help with weight loss or they result in less weight gain. In fact, all of our program participants meet with Dr. Hamdy or another Why WAIT program physician to discuss which medications would be best for them to use to help them lose weight while on this program and keep it off. Since you are doing the Diabetes Breakthrough program at home on your own, you will need to consult directly with your diabetes doctor or another member of your health care team to get help with making appropriate adjustments to your medications.

Talk with Your Health Care Provider about Your Medications

The diabetes medication adjustments that Dr. Hamdy and his colleagues use for the Why WAIT program participants have been included for you and your health care team's convenience in Appendix E. The table that follows also gives you an overview of which medications are generally more weight-friendly or that at least won't make you gain more weight.

Given that it is one of the most widely prescribed medications for people with type 2 diabetes, it is fortunate that metformin (brand name Glucophage) does not cause weight gain. If you are taking it, you don't need to worry about changing to another medication to lose weight. However, if you take a sulfonylurea like glyburide (which is sold as various brand names), glipizide (Glucotrol), or glimepiride (Amaryl) or an insulin sensitizer like Actos, talk to your provider about possibly stopping those medications or reducing your doses. You may want to replace them with one of the newer medications called DPP-4 inhibitors, which currently include Januvia, Onglyza, Tradjenta, Nesina (in the U.S.A.) and Galvus (in Europe), or use other medications called SGLT-2 inhibitors, which currently include Invokana (in the U.S.A.), Farxiga (U.S.A.), Forxiga (in Europe and Canada) and Jardiance. None of these cause weight gain. Injectable medications, which are called GLP-1 receptor agonists like Byetta, Bydureon, Victoza, Trulicity, Tanzeum (U.S.A.) and Eperzan (Europe) and Lyxumia actually enhance weight loss. However, be forewarned that these newer medications are more expensive and may not be covered by your insurance.

If you currently take Lantus, Humulin N or Novolin N, we suggest that you discuss with your doctor the possibility of switching to Levemir to cover your basal insulin needs instead. Although all of these insulins can cause weight gain, Levemir generally results in less weight gain than the others.

If you take any short-acting insulin to cover your meals and other food intake, including Humalog, NovoLog or Apidra, you may want to inject this insulin immediately after a meal instead of before or within 20 minutes after you start eating. When you inject insulin based on what you actually ate rather than on what you think you will, you may be able to reduce your insulin dose or eat less. If you're taking short-acting insulin before a meal and get full before you're finished with what you planned to eat (and dosed for), you'll likely keep eating anyway due to fear of low blood glucose. Without that to worry about, you can eat less and only dose with exactly what you need after you finish. Check with your diabetes doctor before changing insulin dose or time of injection, however.

MEDICATIONS TO BE REDUCED OR STOPPED TO ALLOW FOR OPTIMAL WEIGHT LOSS (Weight Fury: Cause Weight Gain) (-)	MEDICATIONS TO BE ADDED OR USED TO REPLACE OTHERS THAT CAUSE WEIGHT GAIN (Weight-Friendly or Weight Neutral) (+)
Sulfonylureas Micronase, Diabeta, Glynase (glyburide), Glibenclamide (outside U.S.A.) Glucotrol (glipizide) Amaryl (glimepiride) Diamicron, Glizid, Glyloc, Reclide (gliclazide, outside U.S.A. only)	**Metformin** Glucophage, Glumetza, Fortamet (metformin) Glucophage XR (metformin ER)
Glinides (Meglitinides) Starlix (nateglinide) Prandin, NovoNorm (repaglinide)	**DPP-4 inhibitors** Januvia (sitagliptin) Onglyza (saxagliptin) Tradjenta (linagliptin) Nesina (alogliptin) Galvus (vildagliptin, outside U.S.A. only) **SGLT-2 inhibitors** Invokana (canagliflozin) Farxiga/Forxiga (dapagliflozin) Jardiance (empagliflozin)
Thiazolidinediones (TZDs) Actos (pioglitazone) Avandia (rosiglitazone)	**GLP-1 receptor agonists** Byetta (exenatide) Bydureon (exenatide extended release) Victoza (liraglutide) Trulicity (dulaglutide) Tanzeum/Eperzan (albiglutide) Lyxumia (lixisenatide)

Insulins	Insulins
Long-Acting	**Long-Acting**
Humulin N, Novolin N (NPH)	Levemir (detemir)
Humulin R, Novolin R (regular insulin)	Tresiba (degludec)
Lantus (glargine), Toujeo (glargine U-300)	
Insulins	**Insulins**
Short-Acting (pre-meal injection)	**Short-Acting (post-meal injection)**
NovoLog (aspart, aspart 70/30)	NovoLog (aspart, aspart 70/30)
Humalog (lispro, lispro 75/25)	Humalog (lispro, lispro 75/25)
Apidra (glulisine)	Apidra (glulisine)
Inhaled Insulin	**Amylin analog**
Afrezza	Symlin (pramlintide)
	Alpha-glucosidase inhibitors
	Precose, Glucobay (acarbose)
	Glyset (miglitol)
	Colesevelam
	Welchol (colesevelam)
	Bromocriptine
	Cycloset (bromocriptine)

Changing medications to promote weight loss or to at least keep you from gaining any more weight is a key decision, but it's equally important to make sure that your doses of any medications are appropriately lowered as you start to lose weight and need less of them to manage your blood glucose levels. Contact your provider to assist you with dose reduction, particularly if you start having more frequent episodes of low blood glucose. Have all your blood glucose numbers ready to share when making these important joint decisions about managing your diabetes.

PREVENT LOW BLOOD GLUCOSE CAUSED BY MEDICATIONS

You may be worried about getting low blood glucose, which can happen more easily when you cut your calories and lose some weight. Generally, if your blood glucose control is within a reasonable range, you may safely reduce any insulin you take for meals (Humalog, Novolog, Apidra, regular insulin or Afrezza) by 20 to 30 percent to prevent low blood glucose. As weight continues to go down, you may need to also reduce long-acting insulins like glargine (Lantus, Toujeo), detemir (Levemir) or NPH. You should communicate with your doctor to make these adjustments.

If you inject pramlintide (Symlin), you should also take it at the right time before meals to prevent lows most effectively. It frequently reduces your appetite, so you may end up eating less than what you plan to eat. Injecting Symlin before eating and short-acting insulin immediately after a meal or within 20 minutes from the start of the meal may be a good strategy. In this scenario, you will inject based on what you already ate and not on what you are assuming to eat since you may not eat it. We noticed that many people continue to eat after they are full for the fear of getting low blood sugar because they injected too much insulin based on wrong assumption before the meal when they were hungry. Basically, they are feeding the insulin and not themselves and consequently gain more weight.

During weight loss, you'll need to closely monitor your blood glucose, though—at least four to six times a day for a while, including before each meal, sometimes two to three hours after eating, before and after exercise sessions and at bedtime. If you take insulin alone or with Symlin, you'll need to check again two to three hours afterward to prevent lows, because the more you have to treat with extra glucose or food intake, the harder it will be for you to lose weight (since all the calories count).

HOW DIABETES PILLS WORK

Your physician may have prescribed one or more pills to help you control your blood glucose by different means and to manage your weight. Some oral diabetes medications work by helping the pancreas produce more insulin. These medications fall into one of two groups: sulfonylureas, such as glyburide (Diabeta, Micronase), glipizide (Glucotrol and Glucotrol XL), glimepiride (Amaryl) and glinides like repaglinide (Prandin) and nateglinide (Starlix). Their downside is that they can potentially cause your blood glucose to get too low, ultimately causing weight gain when you have to treat bouts of hypoglycemia. Although these medications are cheap and very effective in lowering blood glucose, their stimulation of insulin production generally leads to weight gain.

Pills like pioglitazone (Actos) help the cells in your muscles and liver become more sensitive to insulin so that they work better. Another one from the same group, Avandia (rosiglitazone), is rarely prescribed nowadays because of concerns that its use may be associated with an increased risk of having a heart attack, although the FDA recently revised that to a lesser warning, based on new research findings. While these medications don't cause hypoglycemia, their major side effect is weight gain.

Other pills including the commonly used metformin (Glucophage) improve your body sensitivity to insulin and decrease the amount of glucose released by the liver, while others like acarbose (Precose) and miglitol (Glyset) decrease the absorption of carbohydrates in the intestines. These medications don't cause hypoglycemia or weight gain.

Some newer oral medications have combined actions that help your body produce the right amount of insulin at the right time and decrease the release of glucose from the liver, including sitagliptin (Januvia), saxagliptin (Onglyza), linagliptin (Tradjenta), alogliptin (Nesina) and vildagliptin (Galvus, approved for use outside the United States only). These are the so-called DPP-4 inhibitors, which in general don't cause hypoglycemia or weight gain.

Other newer medications include bromocriptine (Cycloset), which works on the brain and colesevelam (Welchol), which combines with the bile in the intestine. These medications have vague mechanisms by which they work, but definitely don't cause hypoglycemia or weight gain.

Finally, the newest class of medications called SGLT-2 inhibitors neither stimulates the pancreas nor improves insulin sensitivity; rather, it works on the kidneys to prevent recycling of glucose back to the body so that excess glucose in the bloodstream spills into the urine and gets removed (thereby lowering your blood glucose levels). These medications include canagliflozin (Invokana), dapagliflozin (Farxiga/Forxiga), and empagliflozin (Jardiance). These medications don't cause hypoglycemia, but help reduce body weight by causing the loss of some glucose calories in the urine. It's likely that many others from this class of medications will be approved for use over the next few years (including empagliflozin, ipragliflozin, tofogliflozin, sergliflozin and remogliflozin), given their dual benefits on blood glucose and body weight.

As mentioned, you'll need to contact your health care team to help you make adjustments to your medications to help you lose weight and reduce your doses as you lose weight. Also, keep in mind that following a meal plan and doing regular physical activity are as important to managing your blood glucose levels as taking pills and doing both together gives you the best result. Injectable medications and some other newer pills that are helpful in controlling blood glucose are discussed in more detail in the next chapter.

TYPE OF PILL	IMPORTANT FACTS	
BIGUANIDES Glucophage, Fortamet, Glumetza (metformin) Glucophage XR (metformin ER) Riomet (liquid metformin)	How it is taken:	Glucophage, generic metformin: usually taken twice a day with breakfast and the evening meal Metformin ER, Glucophage XR, Fortamet and Glumetza: once a day with a meal Riomet: usually taken twice a day with breakfast and the evening meal
	Possible side effects:	Bloating, gas, diarrhea Precautions needed for kidney problems
	How it works:	Decreases amount of glucose released from the liver

GLITAZONES Actos (pioglitazone) Avandia (rosiglitazone)	How it is taken:	Taken once a day Take it at the same time each day
	Possible side effects:	Weight gain, fluid retention Decrease in bone density, especially in women and may cause fractures May cause congestive heart failure in those at risk Cases of cancer of the urinary bladder have recently been reported due to its long-term use
	How it works:	Helps muscles and liver use insulin better (by increasing insulin sensitivity)
SULFONYLUREAS Amaryl (glimepiride) Glucotrol, Glucotrol XL (glipizide) Micronase, Diabeta (glyburide) Glibenclamide (glyburide, outside U.S.A. only) Glynase (micronized glyburide) Diamicron, Glizid, Glyloc, Reclide (gliclazide, outside U.S.A. only) **GLINIDES** Prandin, NovoNorm (repaglinide) Starlix (nateglinide)	How it is taken:	Taken right before a meal, usually breakfast and dinner Prandin and Starlix: taken with meals; if you miss a meal, skip that dose
	Possible side effects:	May cause low blood glucose May cause weight gain
	How it works:	Helps pancreas release more insulin

continued

TYPE OF PILL	IMPORTANT FACTS	
α-GLUCOSIDASE INHIBITORS Glyset (miglitol) Precose, Glucobay (acarbose)	How it is taken:	Taken with first bite of the meal; if you skip a meal, skip that dose
	Possible side effects:	Bloating, gas, diarrhea
	How it works:	Slows down the absorption of carbohydrates in the stomach and intestines
DPP-4 INHIBITORS Januvia (sitagliptin) Onglyza (saxagliptin) Tradjenta (linagliptin) Nesina (alogliptin) Galvus (vildagliptin)	How it is taken:	Taken once daily at the same time each day
	Possible side effects:	Stuffy nose, sore throat, headache, skin rash
	How it works:	It helps the pancreas release more insulin and reduces glucose release from the liver
SGLT-2 INHIBITORS Invokana (canagliflozin) Farxiga/Forxiga (dapagliflozin) Jardiance (empagliflozin)	How it is taken:	Taken once daily at the same time each day
	Possible side effects:	Genital fungal infection and urinary tract infection
	How it works:	It prevents the kidneys from reabsorbing the glucose back into the body, so it spills in the urine

Actoplus Met (pioglitazone and metformin)	Called combination pills
Duetact (pioglitazone and glimepiride)	Two different medicines blended together
Glucovance (glyburide and metformin)	
Metaglip (glipizide and metformin)	May decrease the number of pills you take
Janumet (sitagliptin and metformin)	May not be right for everyone
Prandimet (repaglinide and metformin)	
Jentadueto (linagliptin and metformin)	
Combiglyze (saxagliptin and metformin)	
Oseni (alogliptin and pioglitazone)	
Kazano (alogliptin and metformin)	
Galvumet (vildagliptin and metformin)	
Glyxambi (embagliflozin and linagliptin)	

Adapted from Joslin Diabetes Center education materials.
Copyright © 2013 by Joslin Diabetes Center (www.joslin.org). All rights reserved.

OTHER INJECTABLE MEDICATIONS

Glucagon Like Peptide-1 (GLP-1) analogs include a group of injectable medications that not only stimulate the pancreas to produce a proper amount of insulin in response to a meal and suppress the production of glucose from the liver but also suppress appetite and induce weight reduction. This group includes exenatide (Byetta), which is injected by a pen twice daily within an hour from the meal; liraglutide (Victoza), which is also injected by a pen but only once daily with no relation to the meals; exenatide extended release (Bydureon), which is injected by a syringe once weekly; dulaglutide (Trulicity), also once weekly; albiglutide (Tanzeum in U.S.A., Eperzan in Europe); and lixisenatide (Lyxumia in Europe), also used once daily one hour before the main meal. These medications may cause nausea, but it is frequently mild and disappears quickly. They don't cause hypoglycemia but are the most potent in reducing body weight. These medications can be combined with insulin or any other oral medications except DPP-4 inhibitors. Many medications from this class are expected to be approved in the coming years for their dual benefits on blood glucose and body weight.

WEIGHT LOSS MEDICATIONS

Participants in the Why WAIT program don't use weight-loss medications per se. The medications currently used in the United States are orlistat (Xenical), phentermine, lorcaserin (Belviq), a combination of phentermine and long-acting topiramate (Qsymia), a newer combination drug (Contrave), and liraglutide (Saxenda). Three newly approved medications (locaserin, the phentermine/topiramate combination, and liraglutide) not only induce weight loss, but also reduce A1C levels. Using either of them along with the Diabetes Breakthrough program may improve your results. Talk to your doctor about the pros and cons of all these medications and see if any of them are suitable for you.

Orlistat (Xenical)

Xenical limits caloric intake by reducing fat absorption in your intestines by about 30 percent. In addition to causing weight loss, it lowers LDL-cholesterol levels and may improve blood pressure and glucose control. However, your good HDL-cholesterol may also decrease, and most people experience some unpleasant side effects like gas, diarrhea and oily stools (more likely with the more fat you eat). You can also develop gallstones and some fat-soluble vitamin deficiencies (vitamins A, D, E and K), which would require you to take supplements. The usual dose of Xenical is 120 mg before each meal, although a 60 mg dose is currently available over-the-counter as Alli®. This dose is less effective, but is associated with fewer side effects.

Phentermine

Phentermine is approved by the FDA for short-term use only because its effects are similar to the potentially addictive amphetamine. In addition to having a strong appetite-suppressing effect, it stimulates the nervous system, elevates blood pressure, increases heart rate and frequently causes insomnia. The recommended phentermine dose is 30 mg once daily. This drug is not suitable for everyone and should be used only for a very short period of time, if taken.

Lorcaserin (Belviq)

Belviq is a newly-approved medication for weight loss. It works on the brain to suppress the appetite. Its chemical structure is similar to many commonly used antidepressants, but it works specifically on the eating centers of the brain. The FDA approved it for chronic weight management as an adjunct to lifestyle intervention. It is taken in a dose of 10 mg twice daily. It also significantly reduces A1C levels and blood pressure and improves blood lipids. In general, side effects are mild to moderate but may include headache, upper respiratory tract infection, nasopharyngitis, sinusitis, dizziness, nausea and fatigue. However, be aware that the US Drug Enforcement Administration classified lorcaserin as a Schedule IV drug because it has hallucinogenic properties and users could develop psychiatric dependencies on the drug.

Phentermine/Long-Acting Topiramate (Qsymia)
A second new medication for weight loss, Qsymia, suppresses appetite with a combination of phentermine in a small dose and topiramate (Topamax), commonly used to treat migraine headaches and prevent seizures. Qsymia should only be used as an adjunct to lifestyle intervention. It is taken once daily in the morning to avoid insomnia caused by phentermine. The initial dose is 3.75 mg/23 mg, which is increased to a regular dose of 7.5 mg/46 mg after two weeks, then a maximum dose of 15 mg/92 mg. Side effects include paresthesia (numbness), dry mouth, constipation, upper respiratory tract infection, nasopharyngitis and headache. Topiramate also increases the risk of suicidal thoughts or behavior and mood disorders. It may also cause impairment of concentration/attention, difficulty with memory and word-finding difficulties. It is very important that you not take it if you're pregnant, likely to get pregnant or have glaucoma.

Naltrexone HCl/Bupropion HCl (Contrave)
Contrave is another newly FDA-approved prescription medication for weight loss. It is a combination of Naltrexone, an opioid antagonist, and extended release Bupropion, a well-known antidepressant, and it works by regulating how much food you eat. It is approved for use in adults who are obese or anyone who is overweight and has other chronic medical problem like type 2 diabetes, hypertension, or high cholesterol. It can cause nausea, vomiting, constipation or diarrhea, headache, dizziness, insomnia and dry mouth so increase your dosage gradually. The initial dose is one tablet (8 mg/90 mg) in the morning for a week; increase your dose by adding in a second tablet every evening for another week, followed by two in the morning and one in the evening the third week, and finally two tablets twice a day on your fourth

week. You should only use this medication in combination with a reduced calorie diet and increased physical activity. Don't use Contrave if you have uncontrolled hypertension or a history of seizures, are pregnant or drink a lot of alcohol, and don't take it with other medications unless approved by your health care provider. The antidepressant part of it (Bupropion) may increase suicidal ideations in depressed patients and cause behavioral changes in some people; contact your doctor or a family member immediately if you experience such symptoms.

GLP-1 Liraglutide (Saxenda)

Saxenda, the newest approved medication for weight loss, is another name for Victoza, which is used for treating type 2 diabetes in higher doses. It causes weight loss by suppressing appetite and slowing stomach emptying, hence making you feel full sooner. It has to be injected once a day with a pen (like an insulin pen). Its main side effect is nausea, which usually subsides over time, but it can also cause constipation or diarrhea, fatigue and dizziness. Don't take it if you or one of your family members has a history of a rare cancer of the thyroid called medullary thyroid carcinoma. Stop taking it and seek immediate medical care if you feel persistent and severe pain in your abdomen that might be radiating to your back in association with vomiting.

USE FOOD LABELS TO MONITOR CARBOHYDRATES

Your medications mainly work to help your body process and use the foods that you eat and therefore the more you understand about your diet, the easier it will be to get the most out of your medications. The nutrition facts label (food label) is one place you can find out how much carbohydrate is in the food you are eating and it's important you know that in order to better manage your blood glucose levels. Labels are required to be on most packaged foods in the grocery store.

Nutrition Label

Take a look
at some food labels.

Subtract fiber from
total carbohydrate
if more than 3 grams
per serving.

Nutrition Facts

Serving Size ½ cup (114g)
Servings Per Container 4

Amount Per Serving

Calories 90   Calories from Fat 30

	% Daily Value*
Total Fat 3g	**5%**
Saturated Fat 0g	**0%**
Cholesterol 0mg	**0%**
Sodium 300mg	**13%**
Total Carbohydrate 13g	**4%**
Dietary Fiber 3g	**12%**
Sugars 3g	
Protein 3g	

Vitamin A 80%	•	Vitamin C 60%
Calcium 4%	•	Iron 4%

* Percent Daily Values are based on a 2,000 calorie diet. Your daily values may be higher or lower depending on your calorie needs:

		Calories:	2,000	2,500
Total Fat	Less than		65g	80g
Sat Fat	Less than		20g	25g
Cholesterol	Less than		300mg	300mg
Sodium	Less than		2,400mg	2,400mg
Total Carbohydrate			300g	375g
Dietary Fiber			25g	30g

Calories per gram:
Fat 9 • Carbohydrate 4 • Protein 4

Let's review a few things on the label. "Serving Size" is always at the top of the nutrition facts label. The nutrition information provided is for the serving size that is stated on the label. Remember that the serving size on the label may not be the same as the one in your meal plan or the portion you usually eat.

Next, look at "Total Carbohydrate." Focus on the grams of total carbohydrate rather than the indented grams of "Sugars" below it. Remember that "Sugars" on food labels doesn't differentiate between natural sugars in food like fruit and added, refined sugars, which is very unfortunate. If you only consider the grams of sugars, you may mistakenly decide to exclude healthy foods like milk and fruits while overeating foods like cereals with little or no added sugar, but significant amounts of carbohydrates that will impact blood glucose. Carbohydrate gram counting books can help you estimate the carbohydrate content of foods that don't have a label. You can also access that information online on various websites and using a variety of apps available on smartphones and tablets.

The grams of sugar and fiber are counted as part of the grams of total carbohydrate. If a food contains fiber, you should subtract the fiber grams from the total carbohydrate for a more accurate estimate of the carbohydrate content of a food since fiber is not digested—particularly if each serving contains three or more grams of fiber. If a food contains sugar alcohols, subtract one half of the grams of sugar alcohols listed on the label from the total carbohydrate content as they are not fully metabolized.

SERVING SIZES ON FOOD CHOICE LISTS

The lists that follow show common foods, serving sizes and nutrient content. You can use them as a quick reference. A serving of carbohydrate is equal to about 15 grams of total carbohydrate. As we mentioned earlier, carbohydrate foods turn into glucose in your blood, so it is important to know how many servings of carbohydrate you can or need to eat at each meal. In the Diabetes Breakthrough meal plan, the carbohydrate grams for some snacks and meals are listed, but others are based on choosing an appropriate serving. Learning what portions of varying carbohydrate amounts look like can help guide your choices as you learn how to do more individual menu planning and when you eat outside the home.

Carbohydrate—15 grams of carbs per serving

BREADS, CEREALS AND GRAINS	BEANS	STARCHY VEGETABLES	FRUIT
1 slice bread (1 ounce)	½ cup beans, peas (garbanzo, pinto, kidney, white, black-eyed peas)	½ cup corn	6.5 ounces orange
¼ large bagel (1 ounce)		½ cup peas	¼ cup dried fruit
6-inch tortilla or pita bread		1 cup winter squash	1¼ cups watermelon
½ English muffin	⅓ cup baked beans	3 ounces baked, boiled potato	1¼ cups strawberries
½ cup cooked cereal		2 ounces baked sweet potato	1 cup raspberries
¾ cup average dry cereal		½ cup mashed potato	¾ cup blackberries
⅓ cup cooked rice/pasta		½ cup sweet potato	¾ cup blueberries
2 slices low-calorie bread			½ grapefruit
1 cup soup			½ cup (5½ ounces) mango
			½ cup juice
			17 grapes
			3.5-ounce banana
			1 cup melon
			15 cherries
			1 cup pineapple
			4-ounce piece of fruit—apple, pear, etc.

CRACKERS/SNACKS	MILK	DESSERTS/SWEETS
3 cups air-popped popcorn	1 cup milk—fat-free, skim, 1% milk, 2%, whole, Lactaid®	1 ounce angel food cake
18–20 minipretzels	6 ounces light yogurt	2-inch square unfrosted cake
5–8 regular pretzel twists	8 ounces plain yogurt	2-inch square brownie
6 whole grain crackers	½ cup evaporated skim milk	2 small cookies
3 graham crackers	⅓ cup dry fat-free milk	½ cup ice cream
2 rice cakes, 4 inches across		¼ cup sorbet
17 potato chips		1 tablespoon jam/jelly
10 tortilla chips		1 tablespoon honey/sugar

WHAT COUNTS AS A CARBOHYDRATE?

As you learned earlier, carbohydrate foods get broken down into glucose in your bloodstream. You can help manage your blood glucose by identifying carbohydrate foods and knowing what a single serving is of different carbohydrate-based foods.

What Contains Carbohydrate?
- All plant-based foods
  - Starches such as pasta, rice, cereal, bread, potatoes and legumes (beans)
  - Fruits
  - Vegetables
  - Nuts and seeds
  - All types of refined sugars
  - Fiber (not digested)
- Other foods
  - Milk and dairy products
  - Most sweet snacks and desserts

Let's talk about some examples of foods that contain carbohydrate and which ones to choose. Basically, any plant food can be considered a carbohydrate because some or all of its calories are derived from that nutrient. Carbohydrate is comprised of starch, sugar and fiber.

Starches: Some examples of starches are rice, baked white or sweet potato with skin, beans (e.g., navy, kidney or black), pasta and cereals. Choose starches that are high in fiber, such as whole grain bread, brown rice and cereals such as oats and bran flakes. Check the ingredient list for the words whole grain or whole wheat, which should preferably be listed as the first ingredient. Substitute whole grain products for refined or processed products whenever you can. Use whole wheat pasta instead of white pasta and brown rice in place of white rice.

Sugars: These are comprised of both natural and added source. Sugars are naturally found in foods like fruit, milk and plain yogurt. Many foods also have added sugars, including desserts and soda (considered "empty calories"). Both types of sugar can affect your blood glucose levels, but natural sugars generally are accompanied by many other nutrients, whereas added sugars are usually refined and contain calories, but no or few other nutrients.

Fiber: This essential nutrient is found in fresh fruits, vegetables, whole grains and beans. Fiber is not digestible, so it doesn't raise blood glucose. While it is considered to be a carbohydrate, it doesn't supply your body with energy like other carbohydrates.

Non-starchy Vegetables—5 grams of carbs per serving

1 cup raw vegetables
½ cup cooked vegetables

Non-starchy vegetables include: lettuce, tomatoes, green beans, carrots, onions, broccoli, cauliflower, spinach, cucumbers, peppers, sprouts, asparagus, artichokes, beets, Brussels sprouts, collard greens, kale, celery, cabbage, Swiss chard, zucchini, summer squash, eggplant, jicama, mushrooms, radishes, mustard greens and water chestnuts.

Adapted from Joslin Diabetes Center education materials.
Copyright © 2012 by Joslin Diabetes Center (www.joslin.org). All rights reserved.

AIM TO GET MORE FIBER IN YOUR DIET

We're going to take a few minutes here to talk more about fiber because it plays such an important role in your meal plan. Dietary fiber is found only in plant-based foods and doesn't add extra calories to your diet (unlike other carbohydrates like starches, milk, fruit and dessert). The majority of fiber you eat does not turn to blood glucose. Fiber can't be digested completely because it resists acids and other digestive enzymes in the stomach. There are two types of dietary fiber: soluble and insoluble. Soluble fiber is generally found in foods such as oats, oat bran, ground flaxseed, beans and fruits, whereas insoluble fiber is in wheat bran, apple peel and most vegetables.

Dietary fiber has several health and metabolic benefits. First, it contributes to your gastrointestinal health by adding bulk and helping to move food waste out of the body more quickly. Fiber also helps you feel full and can support your weight loss efforts. Research has also shown that dietary fiber may reduce blood glucose and cholesterol—all while slowing the digestion of carbohydrates to glucose, thereby keeping your blood glucose more stable. A high intake of dietary fiber, specifically cereal and fruit fiber, has been shown to lower your risk of heart disease by lowering your LDL-cholesterol (the bad type). It traps fat and cholesterol during the digestive process and eliminates cholesterol through your stools.

For glucose management and weight loss reasons, the Diabetes Breakthrough program menu plan incorporates 20 to 35 grams of fiber per day, but feel free to eat even more fiber than that if you want to.

Benefits of Fiber

- Water soluble fiber generally helps lower your blood cholesterol and insoluble fiber helps keep your bowel movements more regular.
- Both types also help with weight control and blood glucose control.
- Both types increase sensations of fullness.
- Your daily goal for fiber intake is at least 20 to 35 grams.

HOW MANY CARBOHYDRATES ARE IN A SERVING?

Knowing the difference between a serving and a portion of carbohydrate is important for blood glucose control. A "serving" isn't the amount you put on your plate; rather, it's a specific amount of food, defined by common measurements such as cups, ounces or pieces. A "portion" is the amount of a food that you choose to eat and can be more or less than a serving. For example, a serving of pasta is ⅓ cup. A typical restaurant portion, however, might be more like 2 cups, which is 6 servings of carbohydrates. To understand how much carbohydrate is in a portion, it's helpful to know the amount of carbohydrate that equals one serving (e.g., 15 grams), which is included on the carbohydrate food choice list in this chapter.

What is One Carb Serving?

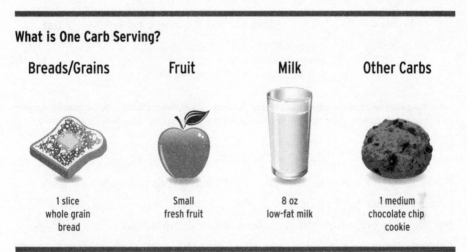

Breads/Grains	Fruit	Milk	Other Carbs
1 slice whole grain bread	Small fresh fruit	8 oz low-fat milk	1 medium chocolate chip cookie

---

COUNT YOUR PROTEIN

Think of some foods you eat that contain protein. A serving size of protein is one ounce of meat, poultry or fish, or one egg—although an ounce of these can vary a lot in terms of their fat content. Alternative protein/meat sources equivalent to an ounce of meat are ¼ cup cooked dry beans (e.g., black, kidney, pinto or white, which are also included on the carbohydrate list), 1 tablespoon peanut butter or ½ ounce of nuts (12 almonds, 24 pistachios, 7 walnut halves, or 7 pumpkin, sunflower or squash seeds). It's very helpful to weigh your protein foods for the dinner menus to determine how much you need and then learn what these portions look like so you can estimate them for meals eaten away from home.

What is One Serving of a Meat/Protein/Meat Alternative?

lean meats, fish, poultry, low-fat cheese	tuna, cottage cheese	beans, peas, lentils (15 grams carb)	peanut butter *
1 ounce =	**¼ cup =**	**½ cup =**	**2 tbsp**

1 serving lean meat = 3 grams fat
1 serving medium fat meat = 5 grams fat
* 1 serving = 2 extra fat servings

As mentioned, protein is a very important nutrient in the Diabetes Breakthrough meal plan. This macronutrient builds and repairs muscle and performs other important functions in the body. What's more, only a small portion of protein turns to glucose. Instead, it suppresses your rise in blood glucose after meals, helps to keep you feeling full and satisfied long after eating and helps you to maintain muscle mass during weight loss. If you eat too much of it, though, it can cause your blood glucose levels to rise about three or four hours after you eat it, particularly if you no longer make enough of your own insulin. In addition, eating too much protein causes you to take in extra calories that you don't need.

Protein: Meat/Meat Substitutes—
0 grams of carbs, 7 grams of protein per serving

VERY LEAN	LEAN	MEDIUM FAT	HIGH FAT
1 ounce chicken/turkey (breast, no skin) 1 ounce white fish ¼ cup egg substitute ¼ cup low-fat cottage cheese 1 ounce tuna (in water)	1 ounce chicken (dark, no skin) 1 ounce lean beef/pork (ham) 1 ounce turkey (dark, no skin) 1 ounce fish (salmon, swordfish, canned tuna in oil, drained)	1 ounce beef (most products) 1 ounce chicken (dark, with skin) 1 ounce veal 1 egg 2 ounces tofu	1 ounce cheese (Swiss, American, cheddar, feta, mozzarella) 2 tablespoons natural peanut butter ¼ cup nuts

INCLUDING FAT IN YOUR DIET

Despite the bad rap that dietary fat has had in the past, it is an essential component of your meal plan. A serving of fat equals 5 grams. Here are some examples of 1 fat serving: 1 teaspoon of trans fat–free margarine, olive/canola oil, butter or mayonnaise (butter is a saturated fat, which is considered to be a less heart-healthy animal fat); 1 tablespoon of reduced-fat mayonnaise, light margarine, 1½ tablespoons of light cream cheese (regular cream cheese is a saturated fat); 2 tablespoons of reduced-calorie salad dressing; 9–10 nuts or 1 tablespoon of pumpkin or sunflower seeds. When eaten in moderation, almonds and walnuts are definitely heart-healthy and you can find other healthy fats in all types of nuts, nut butters, seeds, avocados, olives, olive oil and canola oil.

What is One Fat Serving?

margarine, oil, butter*, mayonnaise*	salad dressing, reduced-fat mayonnaise or margarine, cream cheese	bacon*	reduced calorie salad dressing
1 tsp =	1 tbsp =	1 strip =	2 tbsp

1 serving fat = 5 grams fat
* = saturated fat

The fat servings are already listed in your dinner menus and on the fat list. Learn what the fat portions look like so you can determine what you need when eating away from home. Fat in your diet doesn't get directly converted into glucose so it has a minimal effect on your blood glucose right after you eat. However, it can increase your insulin resistance hours later after it's fully digested when you eat a lot of it—and this can cause a delayed rise in your blood glucose. One benefit of fat intake, though, is that it can help you feel full and stay satisfied longer after a meal because it takes longer to digest.

Fat—0 grams of carbs, 5 grams of fat per serving

MONOUNSATURATED (HEART-HEALTHY)	POLYUNSATURATED (HEART-HEALTHY)	SATURATED (LESS HEART-HEALTHY ANIMAL SOURCES)
1 teaspoon canola/olive/peanut oil 1 teaspoon peanut butter 6 almonds/cashews 10 peanuts	1 teaspoon regular (1 tablespoon light) margarine 1 teaspoon regular (1 tablespoon light) mayonnaise 1 teaspoon corn/safflower/soybean oil 1 tablespoon sunflower seeds 1 tablespoon regular salad dressing	1 teaspoon stick butter 2 tablespoons sour cream 2 tablespoons half-and-half 1 tablespoon cream cheese

YOUR EXERCISE PLAN FOR WEEK 2

This week, you will substitute in another aerobic activity for the one you did last week on at least two of your exercise days (that is, do some cross training). For example, if your aerobic activity last week was brisk walking, think about trying some bicycling, aquatic (pool) activities or some dancing. Doing so will add variety to your exercise routine, as well as give you a lot of other cross training benefits.

WEEK 2: DIABETES BREAKTHROUGH EXERCISE PLAN

DAY	AEROBIC	RESISTANCE	STRETCHING	TYPES OF EXERCISE
1	22 minutes		3 minutes	Aerobic Cross training Stretching
2	22 minutes		3 minutes	

3				
4	22 minutes		3 minutes	Aerobic
5	22 minutes		3 minutes	Cross training Stretching
6				
7				

TOTAL TIME: 25 MINUTES

The Benefits of Doing Cross Training Exercise

- Uses several different activities to reach your exercise goals.
- Adds variety to your exercise program when you include activities like walking, cycling, rowing, swimming, arm bike, weight training, aerobic classes and yoga.
- Gives you flexibility in your program; if it's raining outside and you can't walk, then you can use an indoor bicycle or elliptical machine.
- Reduces the risk of injury as you are not doing the same movement over and over again.
- Minimizes boredom since you're not doing the same exact exercise all the time.
- Uses different muscles during various activities, so more muscles get the benefit of exercise training.
- Makes your daily activities easier on your joints and body.
- Keeps your body challenged to adapt in different ways, so the improvements keep on coming.
- Allows you to rest some muscles so they can recover from workouts without stopping you from exercising (i.e., you can still exercise when injured by doing another activity).
- Helps you develop new exercise skills.

HOW TO DO AEROBIC CROSS TRAINING

1. Choose a variety of activities that you enjoy and include all of them in your exercise program rather than just having a single activity.
2. While you may really enjoy one particular activity, you can actually improve your ability in that activity by adding others that use similar areas of the body. For example, if you like to walk, also doing some bicycling can make you stronger when you walk.
3. Substitute these other activities every second or third day that you exercise, or do different activities with every session; for example, walk half the time and bicycle the other half or do resistance exercise.
4. Substitute as many different exercise activities as you want to.
5. Keep changing your exercise activities to keep you challenged and motivated.

HOW TO PREVENT EXERCISE-RELATED BLOOD GLUCOSE LOWS

It's a good practice to check your blood glucose both pre- and postexercise. If you are taking diabetes pills and Byetta, Victoza or Bydureon, your blood glucose should be over 90 mg/dl when you start. If you take insulin in combination with diabetes pills or other injectable medications like Symlin, Byetta, Bydureon or Victoza, it should be over 110 mg/dl. If your blood glucose pre-exercise is below your target level, take a snack of approximately 15 grams of carbohydrates to avoid low blood glucose during or after exercise. Using glucose tablets—just four of them, equivalent to about 15 grams of carbohydrate—is an easy and effective way to treat lows. If you are on insulin, cut back one to two units of Humalog, NovoLog or Apidra and/or reduce your Humulin N or Novolin N dose by two to four units on days that you exercise.

After exercise, your muscles are using glucose to replenish themselves and continuing to burn calories, which can increase your risk of low blood glucose. It's a good practice to check your blood glucose within an hour of when you finish your workout for that reason. Your risk for developing a low later on depends a lot on what you did and which medications you are taking, but you won't know your risks unless you check your blood glucose levels to find out. At the meal you eat following exercise, you may need to cut back on your rapid-acting insulin dose (if you take that type of insulin) to avoid low blood glucose. For example, if your normal meal insulin dose is five units, you may need to cut back by one to two units for the meal right afterward.

When you begin to exercise at least every other day, your body will also stay more sensitive to insulin for longer, thereby lowering your blood glucose and increasing your risk for hypoglycemia. You may need to check with your health care provider and have him or her reduce your medication doses according to the algorithm given in Appendix E to help prevent hypoglycemia.

How to Prevent Low Blood Glucose with Exercise

- Check your blood glucose before and after the activity.
- Your blood glucose goal before exercise varies based on your diabetes medications:
  - Diabetes pills and/or Byetta, Bydureon or Victoza: over 90 mg/dl
  - Insulin alone, or insulin plus either diabetes pills or Symlin: 110–180 mg/dl
- Eat a carbohydrate snack (15 grams) if your blood glucose is lower than your goal.
- Adjust your insulin doses as follows, based on trial and error:
  - Reduce 10 to 20 percent of the dose of rapid-acting insulins (Humalog, NovoLog and Apidra) for a meal close to exercise; for example, if your total dose is 9 units, you will cut 1–2 units, based on trial and error.
  - Longer-acting insulin (like Levemir or Lantus) may not be adjusted initially; as you progress with your weight loss and exercise routine, you may be more at risk to have a low; talk with your health care provider about possibly reducing it then.

As you lose weight, your need for medication will likely decrease and you may start to experience more lows. One of the goals of this program is to learn how to deal with lows without having to eat more, since even the calories you eat to treat a low count toward your daily total. If you start experiencing low blood glucose more frequently during or after exercise, contact your health care provider as soon as possible to get assistance with adjusting your medications to prevent lows and avoid having to eat extra to treat them.

EXERCISING SAFELY WITH AND WITHOUT HEALTH COMPLICATIONS

As discussed, both your weight control and your glucose control will benefit from regular exercise. But there are some precautions to take to ensure that you are exercising safely. Before you begin, since this program involves exercise that is more strenuous than brisk walking and other daily activities you already do, you should talk with your doctor first to see if you need a checkup or any additional testing.

Remember to check your blood glucose levels before and after exercise; you shouldn't exercise when your levels are too high or low or you're sick. Carry a snack or glucose tablets with you in case you experience low blood glucose. Also, have medical identification (e.g., bracelet) with you and a cell phone if you have one, especially if you exercise by yourself.

Be prepared for the type of exercise you're doing. For example, invest in the right shoes for the activity and dress in layers so that you can add or remove clothing if you need to. It's also important to avoid activities that cause you any pain or that aggravate any preexisting health problems you may have.

If you have any diabetes complications, be aware that you may need to make some modifications for certain activities.

- **Heart disease:** If you have been diagnosed with heart disease, it is recommended that you participate regularly in both cardio and resistance training. Start out at a low level and progress slowly, though, and have an exercise stress test before you start any vigorous activities, since people with diabetes can experience reduced blood flow to their hearts without getting symptoms. If you usually develop chest pain during exercise, keep your heart rate at least 10 beats per minute below where the pain starts. Make sure to carry nitroglycerin with you, if prescribed by your cardiologist and use as instructed.

- **High blood pressure:** Avoid vigorous activity, heavy weight lifting and holding your breath when exercising. Don't exercise if your systolic blood pressure (the higher number) is above 200 mmHg or your diastolic pressure (the lower number) is above 110 mmHg before you start. Taking blood pressure medications can help keep your pressures at a lower level when you exercise, as well.
- **Peripheral vascular disease:** If you experience pain in your lower legs when you exercise, it may be due to clogged arteries there that reduce the oxygen supply to your active muscles. Using pain as your guide, engage in low to moderate intensity walking, taking rest periods as needed.
- **Retinopathy (diabetic eye disease):** You should ideally have a dilated eye exam by an ophthalmologist at least once a year and reasonably close to when you start strenuous exercise. If you have moderate or severe nonproliferative diabetic retinopathy, avoid heavy weight lifting or holding your breath during exercise. If you have proliferative disease (which increases your risk for hemorrhages inside your eyes), avoid doing heavy resistance exercise, running, racquet sports, head down activities, jumping, jarring activities, lifting heavy objects or any activity that elevates your blood pressure a lot. Never exercise with an active eye hemorrhage. Always let your ophthalmologist know about your exercise routine to find out if you should modifiy it based on the results of your latest eye exam.
- **Peripheral neuropathy (nerve damage):** If you have some peripheral nerve damage, you may benefit from doing more non-weight-bearing activities, such as swimming, water aerobics (using water shoes) or stationary cycling, to reduce stress on your feet. Inspect your feet daily for sores, blisters, irritation, cuts or other injuries that could develop into ulcers. It's okay to walk or do weight-bearing activities as long as any ulcers on the bottom of your feet are fully healed, but keep your feet clean and dry, avoid swimming and stay off your feet if you have an infection or ulcer or if you have been diagnosed

with Charcot foot. Always wear appropriate shoes and socks that allow your feet to stay drier.

- **Autonomic neuropathy (central nerve damage):** If you have autonomic neuropathy, it is advisable to have your doctor test your heart's responses before starting an exercise program. You may need to monitor your exercise intensity using the "talk test" (see Week 1). Check your blood pressure before and after activity as you're more likely to develop a low blood pressure and avoid activities with rapid postural changes as your blood pressure may not respond normally (and you could faint). Also, avoid activities in extreme hot or cold weather as you may not be able to regulate your body temperature as well and stay hydrated by drinking water during exercise.

- **Nephropathy and kidney disease:** If you have developed problems with your kidneys due to diabetes, you may have a reduced exercise capacity. Start out by doing low to moderate exercise, but avoid strenuous activity. It's okay for you to exercise daily, though, even during dialysis sessions if you have the opportunity to do so.

Exercise Safely

- Check your blood glucose.
- Know when you should not exercise.
- Be prepared:
  - Clothes, shoes
  - Snacks
  - Identification
  - Cell phone
- Avoid activities that cause you undue pain.
- Talk to your health care provider about exercise precautions related to diabetes complications (eyes, feet, kidneys, heart, etc.).

WHEN SHOULDN'T YOU EXERCISE?

There are times when it's best to postpone your planned exercise to a later time or another day. Before you start working out, check your blood glucose first. We generally don't recommend exercising if your blood glucose is higher than 400 mg/dl, or minimally you should be extremely cautious if you do exercise with it that elevated. Exercising with high blood glucose numbers is not safe when you have moderate or higher levels of ketones, which start building up in your bloodstream when your body is insulin-deficient (which applies mostly to people with type 1 diabetes with inadequate insulin dosing). Be additionally cautious about exercising when you aren't feeling well, whether you have a cold, infection or inflammation. Delay exercise until you feel better, just to be on the safe side.

PREVENTING AND TREATING EXERCISE-RELATED INJURIES

When you start exercising, you'll unfortunately increase your risk of injuring yourself while participating or of developing an overuse injury over time. Take a close look at the causes of injuries, which ones are most common and how to prevent and treat them for the best results. Judicious use of ibuprofen or another anti-inflammatory medication available over the counter can also help control pain and inflammation associated with both acute and chronic injuries. The best medicine is prevention, though. Try to prevent injuries before they happen so that you won't have to take time off from exercising while on this program or later on down the line.

Causes of sports injuries:
- **Footwear:** no arch support, too tight/big
- **Exercise errors:** too much exercise, progressing too quickly with higher exercise intensities, not stretching, no warm-up/cooldown
- **Faulty biomechanics:** high/flat arches, muscle tightness
- **Environment:** walking on muddy, wet, icy surfaces

Common injuries:
- **Ankle sprain:** a painful stretching or tearing of a ligament; inversion sprains are common and occur when your foot twists inward; the outside ligaments are then stretched or torn

- **Plantar fasciitis:** inflammation of the plantar fascia (arch along the bottom of the foot)
  - *Symptom:* pain in the heel when standing or walking
  - *Causes:* shoes with poor arch support, very stiff soles, not stretching after exercises
- **Heel spur:** abnormal bone growth on the heel, which results from untreated or prolonged plantar fasciitis
- **Shin splints:** occur during physical activity when too much force is being placed on your shinbone and connective tissues that attach your muscles to the bone
  - *Symptom:* sharp pain along the lower leg (shinbone) while walking, jogging or aerobic dancing
  - *Causes:* inflammation of the shinbone, stress fracture of either tibia or fibula (lower leg bones)
- **Achilles tendinitis:** inflammation and swelling of a tendon
  - *Symptoms:* swelling, redness, pain, aching, stiffness before, during and after exercise; pain gets worse when walking uphill or climbing stairs
  - *Causes:* tight calf muscle, poor stretching habits, running on hard surfaces and hills, overuse, worn-out shoes

Prevention of injuries:
- Prevention of knee injuries: avoid rapid changes in direction or land from a jump, progress exercise slowly, choose safe activities, always warm up and cool down and stretch your leg muscles on both sides of the joint. In addition, choose exercises that help strengthen the muscles around your knee such as biking, leg press and chair squat.
- Prevention of lower back injuries: avoid heavy weight lifting, avoid rapid changes in direction, choose safe activities, progress exercise slowly, always warm up and cool down and stretch your lower back and thigh muscles

Treating acute sports injuries with RICE:
- Rest: stay off your feet as much as possible and use crutches if necessary

- Ice: cover the area with a towel and place a plastic bag full of ice for 10 to 20 minutes at a time several times a day for two to three days to help reduce swelling
- Compression: use a pressure bandage (like an Ace bandage that you can wrap around the affected area) to help reduce swelling
- Elevation: elevate your foot slightly higher than your heart to help reduce throbbing pain

PLAN AHEAD FOR EXERCISE SUCCESS

In these first two weeks, we have covered some of the details of the exercise component of the Diabetes Breakthrough program. You have learned more about the benefits of exercise, the types of exercise, how to know if you're working hard enough and how to be safe and avoid injuries. Why is all of this so important? The more you know about exercise and how your body responds to it, the more confident you'll feel about being able to make it a part of your life to achieve your goals.

What are some of the things you plan to do to work exercise into your day? One thing that can help you achieve your exercise goals is planning ahead. Look at your calendar, see exactly what your schedule looks like and how you can fit exercise into it and then schedule it in. Maybe Thursday you'll exercise in the morning, but Friday in the evening. If you take insulin, plan ahead in case you need to cut back on your dosage in order to avoid low blood glucose. Using your logbook or calendar, look at the dates and plan exactly when you're going to exercise and what you're going to do. Planning is a good approach to help you stay on track and be consistent—which is absolutely essential while you're losing weight and even more so when you reach your weight loss goal and are maintaining your healthier weight.

Again, remember to listen to your body, which means exercising regularly but also knowing when to not exercise. Avoid injuries by warming up, cooling down and doing some of your stretching exercises. Don't try to push yourself more than you need to on any given day and exercise at a moderate intensity. It's okay to work harder on some days and easier on others if that helps keep you motivated and injury-free. Lastly, be sure to record your exercise in your logbook, along with blood glucose responses and other comments related to how you felt, what worked and what didn't and what you should try next time to get the most out of your activities.

For Exercise, Remember To:

- Plan for success.
- Be consistent.
- Listen to your body to avoid injury:
    - Know when *not* to exercise (such as when you are too tired or ill)
    - Warm up and cool down for 4 to 5 minutes each
    - Exercise at a moderate intensity
    - Stretch muscles after warming up or at the end of your exercise session, which is after cooldown
- Record daily exercise in your logbook.

"DOUBLE DIABETES" NO MORE

You met David at the start of this chapter when you heard about his gradual weight gain and insulin resistance. The biggest issue, however, the one that ultimately led him to enroll in the Joslin Why WAIT program, was that he had developed "double diabetes" (symptoms of both type 1 and type 2 diabetes), causing him to both gain weight and need more insulin to manage his blood glucose levels even though he had type 1 diabetes.

For him, it was a wake-up call to find out that he was now considered not just overweight, but obese. He recalls, "The Why WAIT program motivated me to start exercising again. I lost 30 pounds in 12 weeks and my weight has been stable." Since finishing the program, he has even reconfigured his basement into a home gym—where he has a stationary bike, a NordicTrack machine (that simulates cross-country skiing) and some weights—and he works out daily. The good news is that all of his diligence has paid off. He's thinner again and needs a lot less insulin to control his type 1 diabetes. It's back to well-controlled, "single" diabetes for David now, thanks to the program.

DIABETES BREAKTHROUGH WEEK 3

Portion Distortion, Resistance Training and Newer Diabetes Medications

By this week, hopefully you already know a lot more about yourself and are learning new eating habits and overcoming your barriers to being more active. You should be taking in 1500 or 1800 calories per day—whatever it takes to cut back enough to lose at least a pound of fat every week. This week's discussion will focus more on why people actually eat more than they think they do (portion distortion)—in fact, most people consume upward of 3000 calories a day, even when they need far less—and how you can prevent that from happening to you. You'll also learn more about some of the newer, weight-friendly diabetes medications that you may want to talk to your doctor about possibly using instead to manage your blood glucose levels.

The main exercise focus for this week is on resistance training. While you may be thinking that you don't want to bulk up, we're here to assure you that it's unlikely to happen. You will learn more about how important it is to keep the muscle mass you have, though, especially as you're losing weight and why resistance training is so important for retaining and gaining muscle.

IS WEIGHT LOSS SURGERY THE ONLY OPTION?

Diagnosed in 2005 with type 2 diabetes, Mary's blood glucose had gone up over 300 mg/dl, she was very obese and she had a heart arrhythmia. Her doctor had told her that having a procedure known as bariatric surgery (a weight loss surgery) was the only way she'd ever be able to control her body weight and her diabetes, but she just didn't want to undergo the knife. Having major abdominal surgery certainly isn't risk- or cost-free and close to 3 percent of people who have the surgery require a second operation within 90 days due to complications from the first one. It also can be a very expensive procedure to undergo (in the range of $20,000) and not everyone keeps the lost weight off forever.

Mary isn't the only one who wants to fully examine all of her other options first. We'll let you know what she decided to do later in this chapter (and how it turned out).

GIVE YOURSELF A HAND IN DETERMINING PORTION SIZE

The best part about learning how to eat Why WAIT method is that its dietary plans are designed to be lifelong ones you can easily follow long after the 12 weeks have ended. The program helps you learn how to judge just how much food you're eating and how to prevent overeating in all situations by making sense of portion distortion. All you need to practice is using the hand guide (that follows) to measure food portions at home and when eating out.

There are some easy ways you can keep track of portion and serving sizes. For instance, two tablespoons of peanut butter looks like a golf ball. A cup of rice is the size of your fist. Keep in mind, however, that if you have a big hand, you may have a fist that is bigger than one cup. It is important to figure out how serving sizes relate to your own hands versus the hand of an average woman (1-cup fist size).

The following tips will make it easier to estimate what you're eating. (Note: gentlemen, you may need to estimate down a little bit since your hands are usually bigger than a woman's hand of average size.) Try making a cheat sheet to remind yourself of what an appropriate serving size is. You can check your accuracy by estimating first, then measuring to see if you are correct.

Hand Guide to Sensible Servings

Your fist . . . is about the size of **1 cup**
- **1 fist** rice/pasta = 45 grams carbohydrate
- **1 fist** corn/peas/potatoes = 30 grams carbohydrate
- **2 fists** potato = 60 grams carbohydrate

Your palm . . . is about the size of **3 ounces** of meat, poultry or fish. Protein servings are usually measured in ounces, so a piece of grilled chicken breast that fits in the palm of your hand counts as "3 protein servings."

Your thumb . . . is about the size of **1 ounce** of cheese or **1 tablespoon** of salad dressing or peanut butter.

Your thumb tip (the top joint of your thumb) . . . is about **1 teaspoon.** One teaspoon equals one serving of fat, such as margarine, mayonnaise or oil.

Picture These Sensible Servings When You're Eating Out

1 ounce of meat or cheese
looks like a matchbook

3 ounces of meat
looks like a deck of cards

1 tablespoon of peanut butter
is the size of a walnut

1 cup of fruit, green salad
or frozen yogurt is the size
of a baseball

A medium apple or orange or $1/2$ cup
of low-fat ice cream or yogurt is
about the size of a tennis ball

A bunch of grapes equal
to a $1/2$ cup serving is about
the size of a light bulb

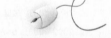

A medium potato is about
the size of a computer mouse

When It Comes to Portion Sizes, Remember . . .

- Using measuring cups and a kitchen scale is the best way to keep close tabs on your portion sizes and your blood glucose levels.
- With practice, you'll be able to estimate accurately and you will not need to use the cups or the scale all the time.
- When you eat out a lot, your idea of a serving tends to increase without your noticing. When you're at home, it is always a good idea to check your portions and keep your portion estimation skills strong.

MAKE SENSE OF PORTION DISTORTION

The amount of food you eat affects your blood glucose levels and controlling portions of all foods helps manage your body weight, as well. You have the power to overcome portion distortion by practicing portion control. So why do so many of us have problems with controlling portion size? There are several reasons, starting with the three C's:

Convenience: Eating at restaurants can make controlling portions difficult. It can be convenient to get food from a restaurant, but most portions are too large. For example, fast food meals and drive-through windows are easy and convenient, but portions are often "supersized."

Cost: It is often more economical to get a larger amount of some food than a smaller amount for the same price (like a "value meal" or "dollar menu") and we are attracted by the idea of getting "more bang for our buck." Likewise, all-you-can-eat buffets may be cost-effective, but eating at them makes it almost impossible to control your food intake.

Current lifestyle: Forty percent of meals that Americans consume are eaten out. You will soon realize how hard it is to stay on track with your weight management if you frequently eat at restaurants. Eating out used to be a treat reserved for special occasions, but now it is an ordinary, everyday occurrence. You can't "treat" yourself two or three times a day by eating out and think that you'll still be able to achieve your weight loss and blood glucose goals.

Remember that learning to control portion size is vital to successful weight loss and maintenance because it affects the balance of calories in and calories out. When you eat out, use those handy references for estimating appropriate portion sizes based on your target calorie intake. Write down the hand references and the sensible serving visual cues references on a piece of paper and carry them with you to use when dining out. Also, if you have been using the dinner menus at home, use them as a template to build on when dining out.

You should also be thinking about how much activity is required to burn the extra calories in today's generally larger serving sizes. Plan to incorporate some of these ideas for controlling portion size and burning more calories into your new healthy lifestyle.

Strategies for Portion Control

- Use the hand method—measure food portions at home and use hands as reference tools to estimate food portions when you dine out.
- Make guesstimates on portions based on your measurements at home so that you will be able to make a more informed decision on how much you are going to eat.
- Learn visual cues, such as 2 tablespoons of peanut butter looks like a golf ball on a spoon or 6 ounces of meat is the size of two decks of cards.
- Check serving sizes and how many servings are in a package before you decide how many servings you are allowed in your plan; one serving is not necessarily what you should or should not have.
- Use the balanced plate method—⅓ carbohydrates, ⅓ protein/fat, ⅓ vegetables.

WHY EATING NORMAL PORTIONS HAS GOTTEN HARDER

Have you noticed how fast-food portion sizes have increased over the years? Just consider the difference in the portion size of a small order of French fries 20 years ago and today. How many calories would you guess is in today's portion? A small order used to be 2.4 ounces and only 210 calories, but today's portion is 7 ounces and 610 calories. That's a 400-calorie difference compared with just two decades ago.

How long do you think you would need to walk at a leisurely pace in order to burn the extra 400 calories in today's serving of fries? Walking at a leisurely pace (2 miles per hour), it would take a woman weighing 260 pounds, 1 hour and 53 minutes to burn off the extra 400 calories.

It's not just fast foods like fries that have increased in size. Twenty years ago, a typical bagel was three inches in diameter, but now it's at least twice that size. Today's average bagel has 260 calories more than before. For a man who weighs 260 pounds, it would take 40 minutes of raking leaves to burn the extra 260 calories. But you can fight back. One idea is to request that the bagel be made "skinny," which involves hollowing out the bagel (or you can do it yourself).

You can control how much you eat, even when you eat out, by being assertive when you order. Smaller portions are often not advertised, but you can get them if you ask. For example, at Starbucks, you can get a "short" latte, which is smaller and contains fewer calories than the "tall." Or you could order a side dish instead of an entrée or order a "child-sized" portion.

So you can see why it's important to consider the extra calories that come with today's larger portion sizes. You don't need to passively accept whatever portion size is presented to you, though, as you can always avoid eating more than your meal plan recommends by learning how to estimate serving sizes, even when you don't have measuring tools available.

WHY RESISTANCE TRAINING MATTERS

A recent study in a medical journal, *Diabetes Care*, showed that if you have diabetes, you are likely to lose twice as much of your muscle mass as you age compared to everyone else and that's if you're eating normally. That is a really bad scenario if you want to manage your blood glucose levels and keep your weight under control, because you need more muscle mass to do both.

Then, if you cut back on your calories to lose weight and don't do any resistance training, you are going to lose even more muscle—which is doubly bad for anyone with diabetes because muscle is the largest storage depot you have for the carbohydrates that you eat. However, you can retain your muscle mass if you eat enough protein (participants in another study ate 19 percent of their daily calories as protein) and do resistance training while dieting, because you'll lose more fat and keep your muscle. If you just eat more protein (33 percent of daily calories) without doing the resistance training, though, you're likely to lose more muscle even with the extra protein intake.

USE IT OR LOSE IT

You may be thinking that lifting weights is just not for you, but resistance training comes in many different forms. This program will help you get started by adding resistance training into your life with inexpensive resistance bands that you can use at home and when you travel—without having to join a gym or use them in public.

The importance of including resistance training can't be overstated. Simple, everyday tasks like carrying groceries or getting yourself up out of a chair require muscle strength, which you may be losing as time goes on if you don't use all of your muscle fibers regularly by doing resistance work. Start with resistance bands and then invest in some inexpensive hand weights as well, or just use household items that you can easily lift (like water bottles or canned food).

Many different types of training come under the umbrella of resistance training. Although we haven't introduced you to all of them yet (e.g., superset training), you'll be familiar with them all by the end of this 12-week program. Mix them up on any given day or week to get the most out of your training.

Your Exercise Program

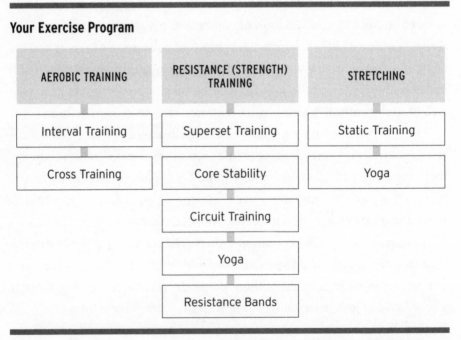

AEROBIC TRAINING	RESISTANCE (STRENGTH) TRAINING	STRETCHING
Interval Training	Superset Training	Static Training
Cross Training	Core Stability	Yoga
	Circuit Training	
	Yoga	
	Resistance Bands	

RESISTANCE TRAINING IS FOR MORE THAN BULKING UP

Women have less muscle mass and more body fat than men, making resistance training even more important for them as a means to change their body composition for the better—which also helps with blood glucose metabolism and burning more calories on a daily basis. Getting "bulked up" from resistance training is unlikely to happen to you if you're female because women are lacking the high levels of testosterone that men have that promote significant muscle gains. As a woman, your muscles will simply become more toned, your waist and hips will get slimmer and you'll lose inches instead.

When people lose weight, they often lose muscle along with fat. Losing muscle can cause your metabolism to drop, which will in turn make it more difficult for you to continue to lose weight or keep your diabetes in control. Resistance exercise helps maintain or even increase your muscle mass, which is the main place your body stores any excess carbohydrates that you eat.

Normally when you exercise, your liver releases enough glucose to keep your blood levels optimal. The glucose travels through the bloodstream and goes through the "doors" to enter the muscle cells. Resistance training causes your muscles to use more glucose during exercise and more fat at rest, the result being that you'll be burning more calories overall and will get better results from your weight loss program. Having more muscle also means you'll burn more calories doing anything. It's vital for women in particular to incorporate resistance training into their exercise plan.

Facts about Muscles

- With training, your muscles' ability to burn fat at rest increases.
- Trained muscles store more glucose (as glycogen) and fat than untrained muscles, giving you a greater storage capacity.
- Muscle is more dense than fat, so you can lose inches even if your weight doesn't change with resistance training.
- Muscles grow and rebuild during rest.

BODY COMPOSITION AND BLOOD GLUCOSE CHANGES WITH RESISTANCE WORK

Resistance training involves working against weight, force or gravity. Working against resistance builds muscle, which burns more calories than fat on a daily basis, so having more muscle increases metabolism. Muscle is also denser than fat, so you may not see a change on the scale, but you are likely to experience looser-fitting clothes. That's why it's important to measure your success in this program by not just the numbers on the scale, but on other changes, as well. If you stick with this program, you should see your body fat decrease and lean muscle increase. Even if you can't directly measure those changes, seeing your waist and hip measurements decline will let you know you're losing fat while increasing your muscle mass and toning and strengthening your muscles.

Facts about Resistance Training

- Involves working against weight, force or gravity.
- Increases muscle size (hypertrophy).
- Maintains high speed metabolic rate for many hours afterward.
- Increases metabolic rate.
- May increase blood glucose initially; however, blood glucose will drop a few hours after resistance training.

With training, your blood glucose may increase at first, but you will probably see a drop after two to eight hours. These fluctuations in blood glucose are why we ask you to check your blood glucose more often, specifically before and after exercise. Talk with your health care provider if you struggle to manage your blood glucose with exercise.

WHAT ARE THE HEALTH BENEFITS OF RESISTANCE TRAINING?

There really is no end to the benefits of resistance training to your health—especially if you want to live a long, healthy and independent life. The benefits of resistance training include increasing metabolic rate, reducing body fat, burning glucose and building stronger muscles. Due to the stress of the muscle pulling on the bone, resistance training has also been shown to build stronger bones. And, as mentioned, it changes the appearance of your muscles, making you look more toned and fit instead of flabby and out of shape. Resistance training is also beneficial in protecting your joints and preventing injuries by strengthening the muscles around them and it also improves your posture.

Resistance training involves repetitive muscle contractions that increase the transport of glucose into the cells. This leads to higher sensitivity to insulin and better blood glucose control, which can decrease your need for medications—one reason that you may need to ask your health care provider about making adjustments to your medication as you increase your activity levels during the program.

Benefits of Resistance Training
- Increases metabolism.
- Burns stored fat and glucose.
- Helps with weight loss.
- Reduces insulin resistance.
- Improves blood glucose control and A1C.
- Increases muscle strength and mobility.
- Reduces the need for medications.
- Increases bone density.
- Tones your muscles (you look better).
- Improves your posture.
- Raises your mood and state of mind.

RESISTANCE TRAINING OPTIONS

You have many different options for resistance training, including using resistance machines, free weights or resistance bands. Since there are a variety of ways to do this kind of training, you can choose what works best for you. Your choice doesn't really matter, just as long as you stick with your exercise

...ange your routine for variety as long as you do the appropri-
...tal exercises and work out around the same number of days
...act, it's probably better to keep your routine varied so that
you're not always doing the same thing over and over. It's also important to
make progress in terms of your resistance, either by using heavier weights or
by increasing the number of repetitions and sets. Resistance training should
now be part of your plan, so include what you do each week in your logbook.

MUSCLE TRAINING BASICS

It's possible to choose from a number of resistance exercises to work the same
muscle groups and you are welcome to choose the ones that work best for
you—given your preferences and any possible limitations. Keep in mind that
almost all resistance work can be done sitting instead of standing.

You should include exercises that work both your upper and lower body
and core muscles in your torso. Include several exercises each for your back,
chest, arms, shoulders, legs and abdominal and low back areas. Always work
the muscle groups on both sides of a joint, such as the front (biceps) and back
(triceps) of your upper arm, not just one side. All lower body and core exercises
also help improve your balance, which is important to work on as you get older.

Muscle Groups

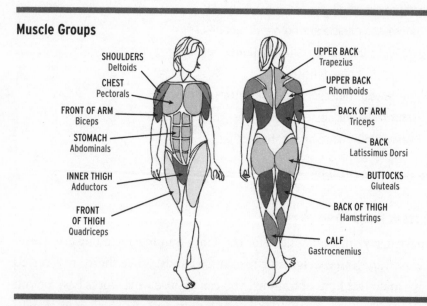

SHOULDERS
Deltoids

CHEST
Pectorals

FRONT OF ARM
Biceps

STOMACH
Abdominals

INNER THIGH
Adductors

FRONT
OF THIGH
Quadriceps

UPPER BACK
Trapezius

UPPER BACK
Rhomboids

BACK OF ARM
Triceps

BACK
Latissimus Dorsi

BUTTOCKS
Gluteals

BACK OF THIGH
Hamstrings

CALF
Gastrocnemius

HOW MUCH AND HOW FREQUENTLY SHOULD YOU TRAIN?

You'll start with six to eight exercises that target major muscle groups (that is, your upper body, lower body and core areas) on one to two days per week. The frequency, number of exercises and repetitions that you will perform will slowly increase over the duration of this program until you're up to doing 10 to 12 exercises on three nonconsecutive days per week (alternate days because your muscles need time to recover between resistance workouts). Resistance exercises don't necessarily have to be done with aerobic activity; however, it's important to warm up your muscles before starting resistance training. The best way to warm up if you're not also doing an aerobic workout is to go through the same motions that you'll be using for your workout, but without any resistance. Doing this type of training does count toward your total exercise time on a given day and for the week. It will likely take 30 to 40 minutes to get through 10 to 15 repetitions and three sets on each exercise that you choose to do once you have progressed to that point. Keep in mind that you should feel the specific muscle or muscles really working hard during the last 3 to 4 reps in each set. If you complete the set without feeling somewhat fatigued, choose a heavier resistance or weight. If you can't complete your goal number of reps, try using a lighter amount. Make sure to take time to stretch any muscles that feel tight during workouts, since that will help with increasing both your flexibility and your strength.

Resistance Training: How Much and How Often?
- 2-3 sets per exercise.
- 10-15 repetitions per exercise.
- *Short-term goal:* 1-2 days per week, 6-8 exercises to start.
- *Long-term goal:* 3 days per week, 10-12 exercises.
- Start slowly and build up.
- Don't do resistance training workouts more often than every other day.
- Gradually increase resistance or weights over time.

PRINCIPLES OF EFFECTIVE RESISTANCE TRAINING

To prevent injury, it's important to perform each exercise using slow controlled motions and a full range of motion. That means you should move your joints gently and slowly through the entire range of whatever motion you are doing, but don't push past the point of comfort. As you increase flexibility with stretching, you'll also find that your range of motion will increase.

Jerky movements can put too much stress on the joint and cause injuries. If you move too quickly, momentum takes over and you lose some of the benefits of working against gravity. Good posture will help ensure that your joints and muscles are in correct alignment and that you are getting maximum benefit from the exercises.

When you are resistance training, be sure to breathe out during the exertion part of each exercise. If you can't perform the exercise without holding your breath, then it's too hard and you need to use less resistance. If you hold your breath, you will increase your blood pressure. Finally, if you experience pain in your joints, stop the exercise you are doing and try an alternate one. There are multiple ways to work each muscle, so it's always possible to find another exercise that you can do that doesn't cause discomfort.

Principles of Resistance Training
- Perform exercises with slow controlled movements.
- Extend limbs and use the full range of motion around each joint you're working.
- Breathe out throughout the exercise, preferably during exertion and always avoid holding your breath.
- Stop exercise if you experience dizziness, unusual shortness of breath, chest discomfort, palpitations or joint pain.

As with aerobic activities, be aware of your blood glucose numbers when you do resistance work and be cautious. If your blood glucose is not in good control or you're not feeling well, you shouldn't exercise. Also, if your blood glucose goes up, do not take a correction dose unless blood glucose is still high one to two hours after the exercise session. If that occurs, you should take a third to a half of your usual correction dose to prevent delayed hypoglycemia. If your blood glucose is below your target, have a snack.

YOUR EXERCISE PLAN FOR WEEK 3

While your training program is similar to last week by having both aerobic and cross training exercise included (as you desire), notice that your total time increases by five minutes per training day. In addition, you'll really get started on doing some resistance training this week, which you will include as part of your exercise plan from here on out—hopefully at least one to two nonconsecutive days to start this week, with an ultimate goal of three to four days per week as you progress. Luckily, your resistance work counts toward your total exercise time on any given day, so you won't really be required to come up with a lot of extra time to fit it in.

WEEK 3: DIABETES BREAKTHROUGH EXERCISE PLAN

DAY	AEROBIC	RESISTANCE	STRETCHING	TYPES OF EXERCISE
1	27 minutes		3 minutes	Aerobic
2	17 minutes	10 minutes	3 minutes	Resistance training (2 sets, 10 repetitions)
3				Stretching
4	27 minutes		3 minutes	
5	17 minutes	10 minutes	3 minutes	
6				
7				
TOTAL TIME: 30 MINUTES				

BAND TRAINING EXERCISES

ands come in different thicknesses and colors that indicate varying resistances. To use them successfully, you need to choose the right band
or bands for you. When purchasing a band or package of bands, check their
stated resistance aim to get a range of them (e.g., low, moderate and higher
resistance). Ones with handles are generally easier to use. Use the band with
a door knob as an anchor, or place the band around a very sturdy piece of
equipment or furniture.

Starting out with eight or more exercises that work opposing muscle groups
(such as the front and back of the upper arm) is recommended. Try to complete 10 repetitions in each set and complete two sets per session this week
(with a goal of three sets later on). Work resistance training into your weekly
exercise plan two to three days a week, as you progress with the program, for
best results—either as part of your circuit training or as a stand-alone activity.
Step away from the anchor if you want to work harder.

---

1. **MIDBACK—Thumbs Up
    (or Palms Down)**
    Anchor your resistance band at
    waist height. Facing the anchor
    with a medium-to-wide stance
    and thumbs up (or, alternately,
    palms down), pull your arms
    back and squeeze your shoulder
    blades together. Breathe out
    while pulling and breathe in on
    the return.

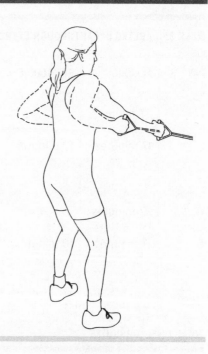

2. CHEST—Press

Anchor your resistance band at shoulder height. Face away from the anchor with a shoulder-width stance and palms down. Press your arms forward while you breathe out. Breathe in on the return.

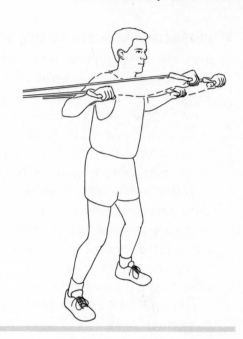

3. SHOULDER/UPPER BACK— Lat Pull Down

With your resistance band anchored over your head, face it with your knees slightly flexed. With palms down, pull your arms down to your sides, breathe out and squeeze your abdominal muscles. Return slowly to the starting position.

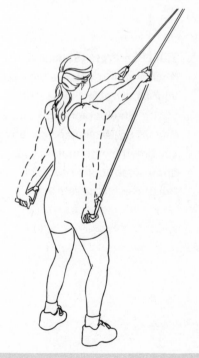

4. QUADRICEPS—Squat (like Chair Squat)

In a shoulder-width stance, anchor your resistance band under your feet. With your palms forward at shoulder height, squat, breathe in and keep your back straight. Don't go past a 90-degree angle with your knees. Breathe out on the return to a standing position. To make this exercise easier to perform, stand in front of a chair. As you bend your knees and squat, your buttocks will touch the chair, then return to the starting position. You can try it without using the band initially, and after you feel comfortable, use the band for more resistance.

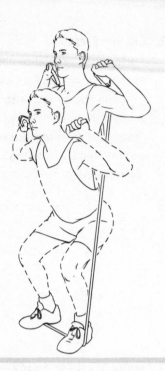

5. TRICEPS—Press (Standing)

Anchor your resistance band over your head. Facing it in a stride stance (one foot forward) with your thumbs up, straighten your arms as you breathe out, rotating your palms down. Keep your elbow joints static. Breathe in on the return.

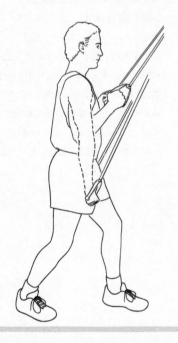

6. BICEPS—Curl (Standing)

Anchor your resistance band under your front foot in a stride stance (one foot forward). With your palms forward, curl your arms and breathe out. Breathe in on the return. To increase resistance, step on the band with both feet.

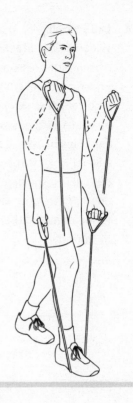

7. SHOULDER/UPPER BACK— Row (Upright)

Anchor your resistance band under your front foot in a stride stance (one foot forward). With your palms down, raise your hands toward your chin with your elbows out and breathe out. Breathe in on the return. To increase the resistance, step on the band with both feet.

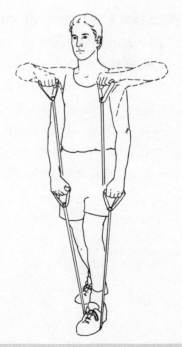

8. LEGS—Walk (Side-to-Side Steps)

Anchor your resistance band under your feet while standing with your feet shoulder-width apart. Bend knees slightly and shift hips backward so knees will not go past toes. Pushing out against the band with the appropriate foot, take 15 steps to the right and then 15 steps to the left.

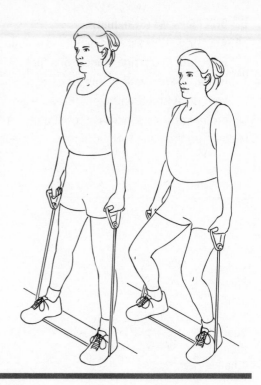

RESISTANCE TRAINING LOGBOOK

Copy the logbook page that follows to use to record your resistance activities whenever you do them. Record the average number of repetitions you do for each of your exercise sets. If you are using dumbbells, barbells, or resistance machines or bands, you will also want to note the amount of weight or the color or thickness of the resistance bands you are using under the "Comments" section. Check your blood glucose before and after these activities and record in your main activity logbook.

RESISTANCE TRAINING LOGBOOK

DAY	SETS	REPS	WEIGHT RESISTANCE COMMENTS
Midback			
Chest press			
Shoulder/ Upper back (Lat pull down)			
Quadriceps squat (Chair squat)			
Triceps press			
Biceps curl			
Shoulder/Upper back (Row)			
Legs (Side-to-side steps)			
Other			

WHAT TO EXPECT FROM THE NEWER DIABETES MEDICATIONS

This week, we're going to discuss more details about many of the newer medications: Januvia, Onglyza, Tradjenta, Nesina, Galvus, Invokana, Farxiga/Forxiga, Byetta, Bydureon, Victoza, Trulicity, Tanzeum/Eperzan, Lyxumia, Symlin, Cycloset and Welchol. All these medications are deemed weight-friendly and may be ones that you want to consider using either now or sometime in the future to assist you with losing weight or keeping it off.

Januvia, Onglyza, Tradjenta, Nesina and Galvus

These five medications are part of a group of medications called DPP-4 inhibitors, which are new pills used to treat type 2 diabetes. How do they work? Your body usually manages to keep your blood glucose in a tight range by sending messages to the pancreas to make more insulin if glucose levels are high and to the liver to release more glucose if glucose levels are low. These medications increase insulin levels when the blood glucose is high after eating and help reduce the amount of glucose made by the liver. In this way, they balance blood glucose levels. As mentioned previously, they are also weight neutral medications.

People with type 1 diabetes, children and pregnant or breastfeeding women should not take any of these. Adults with type 2 diabetes are prescribed a single tablet of Januvia (100 mg), Onglyza (5 mg), Tradjenta (5 mg), or Nesina (25 mg) once a day or Galvus (50 mg) twice daily, as directed by a health care provider. You can take any of these medications with or without food and they may be prescribed for you to use with some other diabetes pills, like metformin, sulfonylureas and Actos, or even with insulin. People with kidney problems may need a lower dose of Januvia, Onglyza, Nesina or Galvus, but not Tradjenta.

Occasionally, side effects like upper respiratory tract infection, stuffy nose, sore throat, skin rash or headache may occur when you take any of these medications. Contact your health care provider if you have any of these symptoms.

If these medications are working for you, your blood glucose levels will be in target range most of the time. Your A1C level will also be lower. When your diabetes is well controlled, your A1C should be less than 7 percent and your blood glucose will generally be 80–130 mg/dl before meals and less than 180 mg/dl after you eat.

Invokana, Farxiga/Forxiga and Jardiance

These are the first two medications available in a new class of drugs developed to treat type 2 diabetes. They work on the kidneys to block the recycling of glucose. Every day around 160-180 grams of glucose are filtered through the kidneys, but they don't appear in the urine because the functioning kidneys reabsorb them back into your bloodstream. This recycling process keeps your urine usually free of glucose. However, when your blood glucose is above 180 mg/dl, it exceeds the capacity of the kidneys to reabsorb glucose and some may appear in the urine.

Invokana, which is approved for use in the United States, Farxiga or Forxiga, (depending on whether you are in the United States or Europe) and Jardiance, are the first three drugs in a group called SGLT-2 (short for sodium-glucose co-transporter-2) inhibitors, which block glucose recycling in the kidneys and cause blood glucose to spill into the urine—leading to a loss of glucose calories (~400 calories per day) and ultimately some weight loss. Your doctor may prescribe one of these medications for you since they enhance weight loss and lower blood glucose. Invokana comes in two doses (100 mg and 300 mg), as do Farxiga/Forxiga (5 mg and 10 mg) and Jardiance (10 mg and 25 mg). These medications can be combined with any other type 2 diabetes medications, but aren't yet approved to treat type 1 diabetes. Since more glucose appears in the urine, taking these medications raises your risk of genital fungus (yeast) infections slightly, especially in women, along with risk of urinary tract infection and dehydration.

It's expected that many new drugs from this class will be approved by the FDA in the coming years since they help patients with diabetes to control their blood glucose and to lose weight. The pipeline currently includes medications with the generic names of embagliflozen, ipragliflozin, tofogliflozin, sergliflozin and remogliflozin.

Byetta and Bydureon

Both of these newer medications must be injected rather than taken orally (by mouth). You inject them into the abdomen, thigh or arm subcutaneously (into the fatty tissue) using the same technique as for an insulin injection. Byetta is usually injected twice a day within an hour before breakfast and dinner, while Bydureon, as an extended release form of Byetta, is only injected once a week. These medications are used for adults with type 2 diabetes only and can be used together with other pills, including metformin, sulfonylureas or Actos. Byetta can be also used together with long-acting insulins (e.g., Lantus or Levemir) to treat type 2 diabetes.

Both work by lowering postmeal blood glucose levels, which occurs because they stimulate the pancreas to secrete insulin. They also promote weight loss by suppressing your appetite and slowing down how quickly food empties from your stomach. When using these medications, you should feel less hungry and eat less, which will likely result in weight loss. In addition, both help lower blood glucose levels by decreasing the release of glucagon (a hormone that stimulates your liver to release glucose) during meals and reducing your liver's release of stored glucose. When first using it, check your glucose levels before each meal and two hours after a meal. You may need to check your glucose at other times until you know how it affects your glucose levels.

Byetta itself does not cause hypoglycemia unless combined with one of the sulfonylureas (e.g., glyburide, glimepiride or glipizide) or insulin. If you experience hypoglycemia when using it, treat it the same way you would treat any low glucose level. To prevent lows, your doses of other medications may need to be reduced. Check with your diabetes health care provider if you experience severe or recurrent hypoglycemia. If you stop taking Byetta for any reason, such as illness or surgery, call your diabetes team before restarting it.

Given that nausea and vomiting are the most common side effects of Byetta, the dose you start on should be low (5 mcg twice daily) and then increased as you can tolerate it without nausea after one month to a higher dose (10 mcg twice daily). If you get nauseous when first using it, your symptoms will usually improve within a short time. Let your diabetes team know if you experience more than mild nausea. To avoid undue nausea, Byetta should be taken no more than one hour before breakfast and dinner. Don't take more than two doses of Byetta in a day even if you eat additional meals besides breakfast, lunch and dinner.

A rare but serious side effect of Byetta is pancreatitis (inflammation of the pancreas). People with a history of gallstones, with very high triglycerides or who are consuming a lot of alcohol are at higher risk for pancreatitis, which usually causes symptoms like severe pain in your abdomen and vomiting.

Unopened Byetta pens are valid until their expiration date. They should be stored in the refrigerator, but do not freeze them. After you open them, Byetta pens can be kept at room temperature (up to 77°F). Once the pen has been opened, it must be discarded after 30 days. Bydureon is similar to Byetta in all aspects, but it may cause less nausea and it has an additional lowering effect on your morning blood glucose levels.

Byetta and Bydureon

- Help the body reduce the release of glucagon at mealtimes, which stops the liver from releasing stored glucose.
- Help insulin to be used properly.
- Help the body produce the right amount of insulin at the right time.
- Byetta is injected 0 to 60 minutes before breakfast and dinner, whereas Bydureon is only given once a week.
- Do not have to be refrigerated after first use.
- Most common side effect is nausea.

Victoza, Trulicity, Tanzeum/Eperzan and Lyxumia

These medications are similar to Byetta in all aspects except that Victoza and Lyxumia are injected only once a day, and Trulicity and Tanzeum are more similar to Bydureon as they are injected once weekly. Victoza can be injected either before or after meals and has the advantage of lowering the morning blood glucose. Similar to when you use Byetta, you should start with the smallest dose possible before trying a higher dose. The higher the dose, the more weight you will lose when using this medication. Trulicity and Tanzeum (marketed as Eperzan in Europe) are both once-weekly injections given with a disposable pen at any time of the day. Lyxumia, which is currently available in Europe, Mexico and Latin America, is used as a once-daily injection before the main meal.

Nausea is also a common side effect and some people prefer to continue on the smaller doses for longer times before moving to the higher dose for that reason. If you have a history or family history of a rare thyroid cancer (medullary thyroid carcinoma), you should tell your doctor because Victoza should not be prescribed for you under these circumstances.

Cycloset

Cycloset is bromocriptine, a drug that has been used for a while to treat Parkinson's disease and some other disorders of the pituitary gland in your brain. Newly approved to treat type 2 diabetes, it lowers your blood glucose without increasing insulin; however, we still don't fully know how it works to control diabetes. It should be taken once daily in the morning (starting with one tablet and working up to as many as six), and it is advisable to take it with food to reduce possible nausea or vomiting. It may also cause severe dizziness that may lead to fainting, fatigue and headaches. Don't take it if you suffer from severe headaches or if you are a female and lactating.

Welchol (Colesevelam)

Welchol helps lower the levels of low density lipoprotein (LDL) cholesterol in your blood, which is believed to contribute to plaque formation in your arteries. Like Cycloset, how Welchol lowers blood glucose is unknown. Welchol comes either as an oral suspension or in tablet form. The suspension comes in packets of 3.75 gm each, and you can take one in a glass of water or diet soft drink with a meal. Alternatively, you can take half the packet twice daily. If you prefer tablets, you may take three tablets (625 mg each) twice per day or six tablets once daily with a meal or liquid. The most common side effects are constipation, bloating, upset stomach and heartburn. Don't take it if you have a history of bowel blockage, very high triglycerides (blood fats) or pancreatitis.

Symlin

Amylin, which is a hormone usually released together with insulin from the beta cells of the pancreas, is deficient in people with type 1 diabetes. Although people with type 2 diabetes may secrete normal amounts of amylin, their bodies resist its actions. Symlin is an injectable, synthetic form of amylin that works to lower postmeal blood glucose and helps promote weight loss by creating an early sense of fullness when eating.

Specifically, Symlin helps slow the movement of food through the stomach and decreases the amount of glucose released from the liver by suppressing glucagon release (similarly to Byetta, Bydureon and Victoza). It should be injected 15 minutes before every meal to heighten your feelings of fullness while eating. If you take rapid-acting insulin with meals, we prefer that you take your insulin immediately *after* the meal to avoid hypoglycemia since you may not eat what you think you will once you start eating. If you start feeling shaky or anxious, begin sweating or feel confused, your blood glucose level may be getting low. Check your blood glucose and if it's 70 mg/dl or lower, take some fast-acting sugar like 3–4 glucose tablets or 4 ounces of orange juice to treat your symptoms.

You have to remember that hypoglycemia is caused by insulin and not by Symlin. To prevent hypoglycemia, your diabetes team will usually decrease your insulin dose by 30 to 50 percent when you start taking Symlin, especially if your blood glucose is reasonably controlled. Symlin is usually injected right before each major meal or snack that is more than 250 calories or 30 grams of carbohydrate. Don't take more than four doses of Symlin in a day, regardless. If you stop taking Symlin for any reason, such as illness or surgery, call your diabetes team before restarting it as you may need to start again on the low dose and increase it gradually.

Since nausea is the most common side effect of Symlin, you'll need to start on a low dose and increase the amount you take slowly. If you have type 1 diabetes, your starting dose will be 15 mcg before each meal and increase gradually every 3–7 days by 15 mcg until you're taking 60 mcg before each meal. If you have type 2 diabetes, your doctor will start you on 60 mcg, which will be increased in 3–7 days to 120 mcg before each meal. If nausea occurs, it usually improves within a short time. Let your diabetes team know if you experience more than mild nausea or if you have even mild nausea that lasts for three or more days.

Symlin and insulin must be injected separately. Inject Symlin into either your abdomen or thigh using the same technique as an insulin injection, but avoid using your arm as an injection site. Also, inject Symlin at least two inches away from your insulin injection site. When first using this medication, be sure to check your glucose levels before each meal, three hours after a meal and at bedtime until you know how it is affecting your glucose levels.

Hypoglycemia can occur within three hours after injecting this medication. Call your diabetes team if you experience severe or recurring lows. Also, you should not use this medication if you have gastroparesis (very slow emptying of the stomach) or hypoglycemia unawareness (low blood glucose without warning signs).

Unopened Symlin vials or pens should be stored in the refrigerator until their expiration date, but do not freeze them. Open vials of Symlin and Symlin pens in use can be left at room temperature or in the refrigerator for up to 30 days. Throw away opened vials and pens after 30 days even if some Symlin is left and never use it if it's cloudy or discolored.

Symlin
- Reduces the release of glucagon, thereby stopping the liver from releasing extra glucose.
- Lowers your appetite when taken before meals.
- Slows down how fast your food leaves your stomach.
- Helps your body use insulin properly.
- Given 3-4 times a day with meals containing a minimum of 30 grams of carbohydrates or 250 calories.
- Most common side effect is nausea.

HAPPY TO AVOID THE SURGICAL KNIFE

Remember Mary and her dilemma related to her doctor telling her that bariatric surgery was her only hope to ever control her weight and her diabetes? We're happy to report that she managed to avoid having surgery and she now has her body weight and her diabetes under good control—despite her doctor's misguided prediction.

How did she do it? She signed up for and completed the Joslin Why WAIT program instead. "I'm so happy I can't tell you," Mary says now, after completing the program instead of having to undergo bariatric surgery. "I really thought I was going to have surgery. I'd been trying so hard on my own and making a little progress, but it was so slow and my blood glucose levels weren't changing even though I'd lost almost 50 pounds."

Why does the Why WAIT program offer successes that people can't always get on their own? Dr. Hamdy and his colleagues recently shared data about why the program is a viable alternative to bariatric surgery. Around 50 percent of the patients who enrolled in the program for 12 weeks and followed for four years were able to maintain an average of 9.5 percent weight loss at four years, while the total group maintained 6.3 percent at four years—still well within the recommended range of 5 to 7 percent weight reduction that improves diabetes control.

Most health care providers have the notion that when people lose weight through intensive lifestyle interventions, the majority gain all or most of the weight back in a year. People have been too pessimistic. They think having bariatric surgery is their only option. But with this program, we are sending an optimistic message: think again. There is something else that can work effectively in the real world and save money, too.

For Mary, the multiple medications she was on before doing the program were the worst and they were costing her a lot of money every month. Why WAIT participants are generally able to cut their diabetes medications by half by the end of the 12-week program, saving them at least $560 a year on diabetes medications alone. "I'm so happy to be on the little bit of medications I'm on now and I'm hoping to get rid of them," Mary adds. "And I'm looking forward to not just the next six months, but to the whole rest of my life."

DIABETES BREAKTHROUGH WEEK 4

Insulin Use, Circuit Training and
Delay and Distraction Techniques

This week we'll debunk some of the myths about insulin use (such as how using it means that your diabetes is "bad" compared to others) and you'll learn more about how different types of insulin work and how to manage them if you have to take any. Your workouts will get a little more exciting this week since you'll be starting some circuit training as part of your resistance work to go along with your aerobic exercise and stretching. We'll conclude with a reminder about why you shouldn't underestimate the power of delay and distraction to help prevent overeating or exercise slips.

RANDOMIZED INTO LIFESTYLE CHANGE

At age 58, Brian is a recent graduate of the Joslin Why WAIT program. He started the program more by accident than by design when he signed up for a research study at the Joslin Diabetes Center. He ended up being randomly put into the group that was given the option of joining Why WAIT to lose weight through lifestyle changes instead of undergoing bariatric surgery—and he couldn't be happier about it. We'll tell you later why it worked so well for him and why he's so happy.

LEARN MORE ABOUT INSULIN

Insulin is an injectable hormone that greatly lowers blood glucose, can help people with type 2 diabetes reach blood glucose targets and is required by all individuals with type 1 diabetes. Some people with type 2 diabetes are reluctant to use insulin because they think it will make their diabetes worse, they associate it with complications or they are afraid of needles. It's important to realize that insulin is simply a tool that helps achieve blood glucose targets. Taking insulin doesn't mean that you have failed at controlling your diabetes; rather, for some people, taking other diabetes medications isn't enough to keep blood glucose levels where they should be. Insulin can lower your blood glucose levels and help you feel better when they have been consistently too high.

There are several types of insulin and each has a certain time period over which it works (generally from two hours to over 24 hours). Some are taken to cover your basal (daily) insulin needs and have a longer duration of action, whereas you may need to inject others for each meal or snack to cover the blood glucose arising from the food that you eat for the next two or three hours. Many of the newer insulins (like Humalog, NovoLog and Apidra) are actually insulin analogs instead of recombinant human insulin, meaning that their physical structures have been slightly altered to modify their action, peak and/or duration of action. In order to understand how the insulin is going to work in your body, it's helpful to know the onset, peak and duration of the insulin you take.

- **Onset** refers to when the insulin starts to work.
- **Peak** refers to when the insulin works hardest.
- **Duration** refers to how long the insulin works.

Usual Actions of Insulin by Type

	TYPE	TIMING	ONSET	PEAK	DURATION
Rapid-Acting	**Humalog** (lispro) **NovoLog or NovoRapid** (aspart) **Apidra** (glulisine **Afrezza** (inhaled insulin)	0–15 minutes before meal	10–30 minutes	30 minutes– 3 hours	3–5 hours

Short-Acting	Humulin R, Novolin R (human regular insulin)	30 minutes before meal	30-60 minutes	2-5 hours	Up to 12 hours
Intermediate-Acting	Humulin N, Novolin N (NPH, or human insulin isophane)	Does not need to be taken with meal	90 minutes-4 hours	4-12 hours	Up to 24 hours
Long-Acting	Lantus, Toujeo (glargine) Levemir (detemir)	Does not need to be taken with meal	45 minutes-4 hours	Minimal	Up to 24 hours
Ultra-Long-Acting	Tresiba (degludec) Ryzodeg (degludec plus glulisine)	Does not need to be taken with meal, but should be	30 minutes-90 minutes	None	Over 24 hours

You are more likely to have low blood glucose when your insulin is peaking, during periods of increased physical activity or if you are eating less food. Once you start this program, your body may need less insulin because of your food intake and activity levels. If you are having problems with low blood glucose, talk to your health care provider about adjusting your insulin doses to prevent lows. As you continue to lose weight, he or she may even recommend that your doses of insulin be permanently reduced or eliminated. To make such changes the same way we do for patients going through the on-site Why WAIT program at the Joslin Diabetes Center, refer your provider to the medication algorithm that has been included in Appendix E.

There are several choices for delivery systems for getting insulin into the body: syringes (to give needles), pens (equipped with a prefilled insulin cartridge and a needle, but shaped like a pen for easier use) or an insulin pump, which is a small device filled with insulin that delivers it through a plastic catheter placed under your skin in one spot with a removable needle and changed out every two to four days. If your doctor recommends that you start taking insulin to better manage your blood glucose levels, you can decide then which of these delivery methods would work best for you.

USE OF COMBINATION INSULINS

In addition, combinations of short- or rapid-acting and longer-lasting insulins have been created to allow you to avoid giving more than one injection at a time (since basal insulins like Levemir or Lantus can't be mixed with other ones). For example, Humulin 70/30 and Novolin 70/30 mixes contains 70 percent long-acting insulin (NPH) and 30 percent short-acting insulin (regular); either of these should be injected 30 minutes before eating. Given twice a day before breakfast and dinner, the short-acting portion covers insulin needs for the food you eat while the long-acting portion provides basal insulin coverage over a longer period of time.

Similarly, Humalog 75/25, Humalog 50/50 and NovoLog 70/30 contain combinations of rapid- and long-acting insulins and all three are available as injection pens for easy use. Although injecting mixed insulin twice daily is convenient, it has two major disadvantages: it causes more hypoglycemia and you can't change the doses of either type of insulin separately. The newest combination insulin, Ryzodeg, is a 70/30 mixture of Tresiba and Apidra. It has an onset of 5 to 15 minutes and a peak of 30 to 60 minutes from the Apidra portion of the dose (given to cover a meal), but an overall duration of more than 24 hours.

YOUR EXERCISE PLAN FOR WEEK 4

While your training program is similar to last week's by having both aerobic (cross training) and resistance training exercise included (as you desire), notice that your total time increases by ten minutes per training day. In addition, you'll really get started on doing some circuit training this week, which you will include as part of your exercise plan from here on out—hopefully at least one to two nonconsecutive days to start this week, with an ultimate goal of three to four days per week as you progress. Luckily, your resistance work counts toward your total exercise time on any given day, so you won't really be required to come up with a lot of extra time to fit it in.

WEEK 4: DIABETES BREAKTHROUGH EXERCISE PLAN

DAY	AEROBIC	RESISTANCE	STRETCHING	TYPES OF EXERCISE
1	37 minutes		3 minutes	Aerobic, including cross training
2	22 minutes	15 minutes	3 minutes	Circuit training (40 seconds at each station, 2 circuits)
3				
4	37 minutes		3 minutes	Resistance (2 sets, 10 repetitions)
5	22 minutes	15 minutes	3 minutes	Stretching
6				
7				

TOTAL TIME: 40 MINUTES

GETTING STARTED WITH CIRCUIT TRAINING

Circuit training is a conditioning method in which you perform a series of eight to twelve exercises (a circuit) to build both musculoskeletal strength and aerobic endurance. You can use various types of exercise equipment, such as weight machines, free weights, resistance bands, body weight, medicine balls and exercise balls. This range of equipment allows you to target a variety of major muscle groups. Each exercise is performed for a set time (such as 45 seconds) or number of repetitions (usually eight to 15). At the completion of each exercise, move on to the next one in the circuit. Perform each exercise with a limited rest period of 15 to 20 seconds before moving on to the next one. Your goal is to complete two to three circuits in total.

If you don't have access to any of the exercise equipment listed (except for body weight), you can still come up with creative circuits that you can do in your own home using household items (such as soda bottles, water bottles, soup cans, etc.) and use your body weight to do crunches, push-ups (modified as necessary), sit-to-stand exercise, planks, high knees and other exercises that use a combination of aerobic work and work against gravity.

its of circuit training are many. It improves your cardiovascular
vating your heart rate during the course of the circuit, all while
developing muscle strength, power and endurance simultaneously and reducing the time you need to devote to exercise by combining your strength and endurance training into one exercise session. If you pick appropriate exercises, a circuit provides a full body workout that includes upper body, lower body and core body exercises together. It does not require expensive equipment and can be performed at home, either individually or in a group. Finally, it can be designed to accommodate individuals of varying fitness levels and abilities.

SAMPLE CIRCUIT TRAINING EXERCISES

Try out the following circuit created for the Diabetes Breakthrough program, which includes some resistance band exercises. You may want to invest in an inexpensive set of three resistance bands to really make this circuit work for you at home. They're also easy to pack, so you can take them with you when you travel or even to the office to use during the day. If you don't have any dumbbells or small hand weights, grab some water bottles to hold in your hands.

It is recommended that you complete about 15 repetitions or more during each set of an exercise (within four seconds), rest while you transition to the next exercise in the ensuing 15 to 20 seconds and then start the next one. Try to complete at least two full circuits before stopping. Feel free to order the exercises however works best for you, but it's good to consider alternating areas of the body to avoid overworking any of them with two exercises in a row that use the same muscle groups.

1. **SHOULDER—Press (Dumbbells)**

    With your back straight and knees slightly bent, press the dumbbells straight up over your head as you breathe out. Lower them slowly back down to the starting position while breathing in.

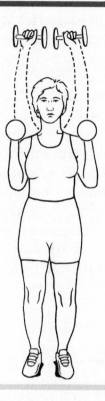

2. **ANKLE/FOOT—Heel Raise**

    Stand with your knees slightly bent and rise on the balls of your feet while you breathe out. Return to the starting position while you breathe in. For added resistance, hold small dumbbells or water bottles in your hands. If you don't have a board, just stand on the floor.

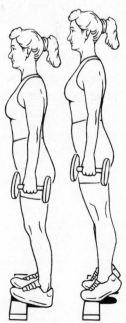

3. LEGS—Supported Squats (with or without Dumbbells)

With your back straight against the exercise ball, which is against a wall, breathe in and bend your knees until you are in a sitting position, but don't allow your knees to go past 90 degrees or to stick out past your toes. Return to the starting position while breathing out. To add resistance, hold some dumbbells or water bottles in your hands during this exercise.

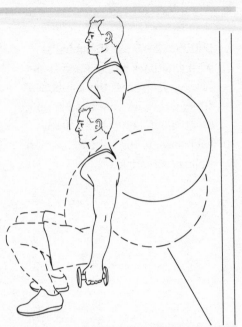

4. BACK—High Row (Standing)

Using a chest-height anchor for your resistance band, face in that direction with your feet shoulder-width apart and your palms facing down (or with thumbs up). Pull your arms back, squeezing your shoulder blades together and breathe out. Breathe in as you slowly return to the starting position.

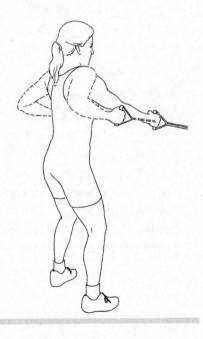

5. TRICEPS—Press (Standing)

Using an overhead anchor for your
resistance band, face the anchor in
a stride stance (one foot forward). With
your thumbs pointing up, straighten
your arms while rotating your palms
down, and breathing out. Return to the
starting position while breathing in.

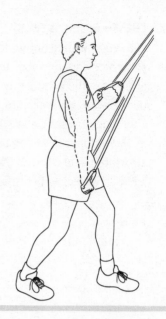

6. LEGS—Step-ups (Forward)

Leading with your left leg, bring both feet up
onto a step (approximately six inches high)
and breathe out. Return to your starting
position while breathing in, leading again
with your left leg. Repeat with your right leg
leading. To add extra resistance when you
feel ready to, hold dumbbells, small hand
weights or water bottles in each hand during
this exercise, or increase step height.

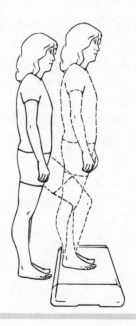

7. CHEST—Push-ups (Wall)

With your arms slightly wider apart than shoulder-width and your feet 20 inches away from the wall, gently lean your body toward the wall until your nose or chin touch the wall, all while breathing in. Pause for one second and gently straighten your arms to the starting position while you breathe out.

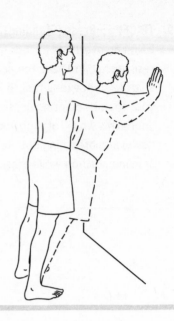

8. BICEPS—Curl (Standing)

Anchor your resistance band under your front foot while you're in a stride stance. With your palms forward, curl your arms up while breathing out and then return to the starting position while breathing in.

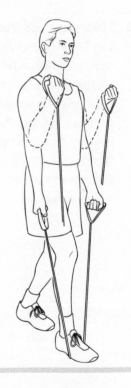

9. LEGS—Walk (Side-to-Side Steps)

Anchor your resistance band under your feet while standing with your feet shoulder-width apart. Bend knees slightly and shift hips backward so knees will not go past toes. Pushing out against the band with the appropriate foot, take 15 steps to the right and then 15 steps to the left.

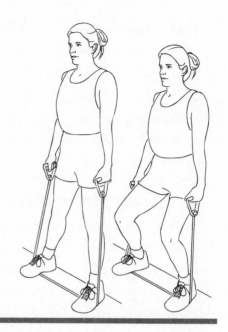

CHANGING PROBLEM EATING PATTERNS

First, let's talk about what you've learned so far from your eating logbook. Earlier, we looked at the ABCs of behavior change to get you thinking about things that have served as triggers to slip away from healthy behaviors in the past. Remember, you learned that the *A* stands for *activating event,* or a trigger, something that might cause you to be pulled off track. We grouped the triggers into four general categories: timing, types of food, activity or situation and feelings. So what are some of the triggers that you identified? Yours may or may not be the same as others you know. Some people have certain times of day when they're least likely to stick to their plan. For example, many people have problems staying on track during the evening. Often people unwind at night after dinner, which can lead to overeating, making poor food choices and not following the exercise plan. Other people have problems when they arrive home from work or while they're preparing dinner.

Once you have identified your unique triggers and their consequences, you can practice defensive or strategic eating, which involves knowing your particular triggers and planning ahead as a solid line of defense. Sometimes this means keeping yourself away from certain foods and certain situations, like keeping high-calorie, high-fat foods out of the house. It may mean working at building a newer, healthier habit such as limiting places and situations in which you eat. Remember, though, that this is a process. You can't anticipate everything. Life intervenes and changes in your plans can arise, in which case you will need to regroup and get yourself back on track. Building healthy habits takes time and practice.

DON'T UNDERESTIMATE DELAY AND DISTRACTION STRATEGIES

When all else fails, do not underestimate the power of delay and distraction to help prevent overeating or exercise slips. You have to find alternative activities for yourself when you know you're at risk. It's important to come up with some activities you can turn to instead of food in order to stay on track. You'll find that with practice some of the items on this list will become new habits that will help you stick to your eating and exercise plan.

Practicing defensive or strategic eating means knowing your patterns and getting ahead of them. For example, consider the following strategies:

Stay away or keep certain things out of sight:
- Keep high-calorie, high-fat foods out of the home and workplace.
- Keep lower-calorie, healthy choices more visible and quickly available.
- Be strategic about what you allow in the house and in your work setting.
- If high-calorie foods must be present, make them harder to see or get to (e.g., use the freezer, keep things stored away).

Build a new, healthier habit:
- It takes time to break an old habit and build a new one.
- Limit eating to one place at home and at work.
- Limit activities while eating; when you're eating, just eat and pay attention.

Your homework for this week is to make your own list of delay and distraction strategies that you think will actually work for you and practice them. You may even discover some new interests or remember some activities that you haven't done in a long time that you might enjoy.

Write down five to ten different activities you can do when you get the urge to eat. (Make sure they are incompatible with eating.) Make them part of your logbook so you can refer back to or update them whenever you need to. Brainstorm about things you can do at home, work and other places you spend time during the day.

_____

_____

_____

_____

_____

_____

_____

If you're having trouble thinking of them on your own, some potential delay and distraction strategies to choose from are listed for your convenience. Feel free to use these or to think of others that are unique to you.

List of Delay and Distraction Strategies

1. Soaking in the bathtub
2. Planning my career
3. Practicing Tai Chi
4. Collecting things (coins, shells, etc.)
5. Going on vacation
6. Recycling old items
7. Going on a date
8. Finding ways to relax
9. Going to a movie
10. Jogging, walking
11. Listening to music
12. Buying household gadgets
13. Lying in the sun (with sunscreen)
14. Laughing

continued

15. Thinking about past vacations

16. Listening to others

17. Reading magazines or newspapers

18. Hobbies (stamp collecting, model building, etc.)

19. Spending an evening with good friends

20. Planning a day's activities

21. Meeting new people

22. Practicing karate, judo, yoga

23. Planning for retirement

24. Repairing things around the house

25. Working on my car (or bicycle)

26. Remembering the words and deeds of loving people

27. Taking care of plants

28. Buying/selling stock

29. Going swimming

30. Doodling

31. Exercising

32. Going to a party

33. Playing golf

34. Playing soccer

35. Flying kites

36. Having discussions with friends

37. Having family get-togethers

38. Riding a motorbike

39. Sex

40. Going camping

41. Singing around the house

42. Arranging flowers

43. Practicing religion (going to church, group praying, etc.)

44. Going to the beach

45. Going skating

46. Going sailboating

47. Painting

48. Doing something spontaneously

49. Doing needlepoint or crewel

50. Sleeping

51. Entertaining

52. Going to clubs (garden, support, knitting, etc.)

53. Going hunting

54. Singing with groups

55. Flirting

56. Playing musical instruments

57. Doing arts and crafts

58. Making a gift for someone

59. Buying music

60. Watching boxing, wrestling

61. Planning parties
62. Doing a jigsaw puzzle
63. Going hiking
64. Writing books (poems, articles)
65. Sewing
66. Buying clothes
67. Working
68. Discussing books
69. Sightseeing
70. Gardening
71. Going to the beauty parlor
72. Reading the newspaper
73. Playing tennis
74. Kissing
75. Watching children (play)
76. Going to plays and concerts
77. Daydreaming
78. Going for a drive
79. Listening to the ball game
80. Refinishing furniture
81. Watching TV
82. Making lists of tasks
83. Going bike riding
84. Walking in the woods (or on the waterfront)
85. Buying gifts
86. Completing a task
87. Going to a spectator sport (auto racing, horse racing)
88. Teaching
89. Taking photographs
90. Going fishing
91. Playing with animals
92. Thinking about pleasant events
93. Reading
94. Acting
95. Being alone (and loving it)
96. Writing diary entries, letters, emails
97. Cleaning
98. Taking children places
99. Dancing
100. Doing sudoku puzzles
101. Meditating
102. Playing volleyball
103. Taking a walk with a friend
104. Going to the mountains
105. Thinking about happy moments in childhood
106. Playing cards
107. Solving riddles mentally
108. Having a political discussion
109. Playing softball
110. Seeing and/or showing photos or slides
111. Knitting
112. Doing crossword puzzles

continued

113. Shooting pool

114. Dressing up and looking nice

115. Reflecting on health improvements

116. Buying things for myself (perfume, golf balls, etc.)

117. Talking on the phone

118. Going to museums

119. Lighting candles

120. Listening to the radio

121. Taking a pottery class

122. Getting a massage

123. Getting a manicure or pedicure

124. Saying "I love you"

125. Buying books

126. Taking a sauna or a steam bath

127. Going skiing

128. Going white-water canoeing

129. Going bowling

130. Doing woodworking

131. Getting a facial or other spa treatment

132. Fantasizing about the future

133. Taking ballet, tap dancing

134. Debating

135. Organizing the closet

136. Having an aquarium

137. Erotica (sex books, movies)

138. Going horseback riding

139. Thinking about becoming active in the community

140. Doing something new

141. Walking the dog

142. Listening to a book on tape

143. Working out with a fitness tape

144. Looking at old photos

145. Sending greeting cards

146. Changing old recipes to healthier versions

147. Planning meals using healthy living cookbooks

148. Joining a book club

Adapted from *Skills Training Manual for Treating Borderline Personality Disorder* by M. M. Linehan (Guilford Press, 1993).

SAVED FROM SURGERY BY THE FLIP OF A COIN

Remember Brian who ended up in the Why WAIT program by accident (most likely with a flip of a coin to decide which research group he should be put into). His weight dropped from 229 pounds down to 192 and, even more important, his A1C went from 8.9 percent to

6.3 percent (from uncontrolled diabetes down to a prediabetes range) in just 12 weeks.

After 12 years with diabetes he'd been taking three different pills and he recalls, "I didn't feel well. It was driving me crazy taking all the pills. I was in denial about needing to change my behavior, though. It took being put into the program to get me to realize how important it was and that I could really do it."

Now he's off all diabetes pills and only takes Byetta, an injectable diabetes medication that helps him manage his blood glucose, eat less and lose more weight. He got his wish, thanks to the Why WAIT program—and he avoided needing major surgery.

DIABETES BREAKTHROUGH WEEK 5

Blood Glucose Lows and Highs, Fitness Benefits and Interval Training

---

This week, we'll be focusing more on some of the daily details of dealing with diabetes—that is, the balancing act to keep your blood glucose levels from going too low or too high. It's important to know the symptoms of hypoglycemia and how to treat it, along with what causes hyperglycemia and why it can be a long-term problem for your health.

Your physical activity focus will be on burning the fat, particularly getting rid of the bad type of fat stored deep within your belly by including some interval training and you'll also be finding out more about what to do on sick days to better manage your diabetes.

DIABETES IS NOT AFFECTING ME (YET)
In her mid-40s, LaTasha has used every excuse in the book for why she didn't need to lose weight or exercise regularly to control her type 2 diabetes. She knew it could cause health problems later on, but she didn't feel that bad now, so she sure wasn't going to spend time worrying about it. Plus, she was young and quite healthy (or so she thought) and the only people she knew that had issues related to their diabetes were as old as her grandfather and his friends,

not anyone her age. Now things have totally changed for her, both in mind and body and you'll find out later how this happened.

WHAT CAUSES HYPOGLYCEMIA?

What do you think some of the causes of low blood glucose could be? Low blood glucose, or hypoglycemia, usually means a value under 70 mg/dl. We mentioned the possibility of developing hypoglycemia a few chapters ago with regard to exercise-induced decreases in glucose. But low blood glucose may be a problem at other times, especially as you lose weight in this program.

What changes are occurring while you are following this program that might cause lows? Some of the causes include eating too little food, having your meal delayed, increasing your physical activity and taking too much of certain types of diabetes medications. Risks for low blood glucose can increase when you're taking medications like insulin, sulfonylureas like glipizide (Glucotrol), glimepiride (Amaryl) or glyburide and others like Prandin or Starlix. Of course, it's also critical that you take the correct amount of medication at the right time.

You can prevent low blood glucose by eating an appropriate amount of food on time, which is why we encourage you to not skip meals or eat less than your meal plan recommends. Your meal plan is designed to keep your blood glucose levels in control while helping you lose weight.

As discussed, knowing how exercise affects your blood glucose is also really important since you have been increasing your physical activity throughout the program. For that reason, be sure to check before and after every exercise session, or at least as often as possible.

SYMPTOMS AND TREATMENT OF LOWS

When you have low blood glucose, you may feel sweaty, shaky, weak, dizzy, irritable or confused, have difficulty concentrating and experience changes in vision, hunger and the sensation of a racing heartbeat. Symptoms can be minor or severe and some may be unique to an individual. It's very important to check your blood glucose with your meter if you ever think you are having a low.

If you experience even a mild symptom associated with low blood glucose, check and treat immediately if your blood glucose is less than 70 mg/dl.

Immediate treatment is extremely important because if your hypoglycemia becomes severe, you can even lose consciousness. Be aware of your own safety and that of others. For example, do not drive or operate equipment that requires your full attention; if your blood glucose is low, do not drive until your glucose levels have risen to above 100 mg/dl after treating it.

How do you treat low blood glucose? First and most important, if you take insulin or another diabetes medication that can cause low blood glucose, always carry some form of glucose or another rapidly absorbed carbohydrate with you. Glucose tablets, glucose gels and certain candies (Smarties® and SweeTarts®) contain straight glucose (dextrose) and act most quickly.

If you feel low, after checking your blood glucose to confirm that it is below 70, follow the 15/15 rule, which is 15 grams of glucose every 15 minutes: check—treat—recheck to make sure your blood glucose has come back up. If your glucose is less than 60 mg/dl, eat or drink a quick-acting sugar equal to 30 grams of carbohydrates, not just 15 grams. While you are in this program, if you experience low blood glucose consistently, contact your health care provider immediately because your medications may need to be adjusted.

Low Blood Glucose Treatment

- Check your blood glucose levels.
- Follow the 15/15 rule: eat or drink some quick-acting carbohydrates equal to 15 grams.
  - 3–4 glucose tablets
  - 1 tablespoon sugar or honey
  - 4 ounces of juice
  - 6 ounces of regular soda
- Recheck your blood glucose in 15 minutes.
  - Follow up with a snack or meal
- If your blood glucose is less than 60 mg/dl to start, eat or drink 30 grams of quick-acting carbohydrates and recheck your glucose in 15 minutes.

WHY ALL THE FUSS ABOUT CONTROLLING BODY WEIGHT?

Americans are continuing to gain weight. As of early 2012, 35.7 percent of adults and 16.9 percent of children ages two to 19 were reported as obese by the U.S. Centers for Disease Control and Prevention (CDC). Other groups have predicted that half of U.S. adults will be obese by the year 2030—a staggering number. Unfortunately, many health problems are associated with carrying too much body weight, including insulin resistance (although you can be overweight and not resistant), high blood pressure, elevated blood fats and cholesterol, heart disease, joint problems, gallstones, fatty liver, sleep apnea and breast cancer.

Recent research in the *Journal of the American Medical Association* on more than 700 participants with obesity showed that people with excess belly fat and insulin resistance face a greater risk of getting type 2 diabetes. We know from various large research studies, however, that losing only a small amount of your total weight (such as 5 to 7 percent) can greatly benefit your overall metabolic health if you have diabetes and prevent diabetes if you are at risk—even if you never reach your ideal body weight or even close to it.

The most likely culprit in all of these health risks may be the combination of a poor diet and a sedentary lifestyle—currently poised to overtake cigarette smoking as the number one cause of preventable death among Americans because together they contribute to weight gain, insulin resistance, chronic inflammation and nutritional deficiencies. The most beneficial way to lose weight and boost health at the same time is through appropriate lifestyle improvements (such as eating more vegetables and exercising regularly) that can be maintained after calorie restriction ends, not from radical or fad dieting.

Weight loss leads to improvements in many areas including insulin action, blood glucose levels, blood cholesterol, blood pressure and inflammation (as measured by blood markers). Doing what you can to retain your muscle mass while losing weight is critical, which you can achieve by including regular exercise (particularly resistance training) into your lifestyle. All types of physical activity also help increase your loss of the bad fat (visceral) stored deep within your abdomen and extra fat in your liver, muscles and pancreas that can interfere with insulin action.

Participants in the Why WAIT program have experienced vast improvements in all of these areas. They have lost an average of 24 pounds after only

12 weeks, which is close to 10 percent of their starting body weights—even while gaining some additional muscle mass—because they've made the lifestyle changes that are critical to losing fat and gaining (or keeping) muscle. They've specifically lost a lot of bad visceral (intra-abdominal) fat, shown by an average loss of close to four inches from their waist measurements and their blood glucose control has improved dramatically, resulting in an A1C drop to below 7 percent (the American Diabetes Association's recommended target) in 82 percent of participants over the course of the program. As many as 70 percent were able to reduce it to less than 6.5 percent (in a prediabetes range). As for their blood work, before-and-after values showed improvements in their blood lipids (e.g., a drop in LDL-cholesterol and triglycerides and an increase in HDL-cholesterol that lowered their heart disease risk), inflammatory markers and kidney function. What's not to like about these amazing results? Yours can be similar if you stick with this program.

WHAT CAUSES HYPERGLYCEMIA AND HOW TO TREAT IT

Hyperglycemia, or high blood glucose, is defined as random blood glucose levels greater than 180 mg/dl. Its symptoms include excessive hunger or thirst, frequent urination, blurred vision, fatigue or frequent infections, but some people can have hyperglycemia without experiencing any symptoms. Checking your blood glucose levels is the most reliable way to know whether levels are high.

Hyperglycemia actually has many different potential causes. Some of these include illness (cold, flu or fever), not taking your medication or not taking enough of it, eating more food than usual, not getting enough physical activity and having prolonged stress (mental or physical). What's more, it can be treated in a variety of ways.

You can try some of these treatment methods when your blood glucose is elevated:

- Take a walk if you are not sick.
- Remember to drink plenty of fluids. People who have high blood glucose often need to urinate more; dehydration can result when high blood glucose makes the body lose water.

- Be sure to take your diabetes medicine.
- Continue to follow your meal plan.

Start checking your blood glucose more often when you get a higher than usual reading. If you have high blood glucose readings for three days in a row, you should contact your health care provider, especially while you're participating in the Diabetes Breakthrough program.

WHY ALL THE FUSS ABOUT UNCONTROLLED BLOOD GLUCOSE?

Like body fat, uncontrolled blood glucose levels can cause serious health complications. Over time, high blood glucose can harm your eyes, kidneys, nerves and heart. On average, diabetes has the potential to rob you of more than twelve years of life while dramatically reducing your quality of life for more than twenty years—through partial limb amputations, chronic pain, loss of mobility, blindness, chronic dialysis and heart disease.

Hyperglycemia can trigger oxidative damage caused by excess free radicals (compounds that cause oxidative damage and inflammation) and the resulting oxidative stress may contribute to any or all of the complications associated with long-term diabetes, including heart disease and eye, kidney and nerve damage. These radical compounds, if left unchecked, promote further insulin resistance and a lower insulin secretion, which is exactly what you don't want to happen if you have diabetes or prediabetes.

WHAT CAN YOU DO TO PREVENT THE DAMAGE CAUSED BY DIABETES?

You may be able to slow the progression of or reverse some of your complications through a little more diligence with your blood glucose and by caring for your whole body. Making even small improvements in your blood glucose control can vastly lower your risk of getting any and all diabetes-related health problems. Diabetes care is rapidly changing and there are new monitoring tools and medications to better control glycemic peaks and valleys and you should have access to everything that you need to manage your diabetes effectively.

How can you control your blood glucose to prevent, delay or slow the progression of complications? Postmeal glucose spikes may be just as important in causing long-term health problems as overall glucose control—maybe even more so. Controlling such spikes may be the key to preventing microvascular complications like damage to your nerves, kidneys and eyes.

Checking your blood glucose not only before meals, but also one to two hours afterward can tell you how various meals or foods are affecting your blood glucose levels and how much variability in your glucose levels you are experiencing. Blood glucose levels typically reach a peak 72 minutes after you start eating (give or take 23 minutes) and both the American Diabetes Association and the American Association of Clinical Endocrinologists recommend checking blood glucose levels two hours after meals. Since most insurance plans won't pay for that many strips for your meter, consider varying the time of day you check your blood glucose instead of always doing it at the same time each day. However, keeping the routine of checking blood glucose in the morning before breakfast is very important. As we mentioned earlier, during the 12-week program, you need to check your blood glucose at least before each meal and at bedtime since you may change your medication dose as you lose weight.

Since the majority of diabetes-related complications are also likely related to unchecked oxidative stress in various tissues and organs, eating foods containing more natural antioxidant power, such as blueberries and sweet potatoes, may help to prevent some of the potentially negative impact of elevated blood glucose. Interestingly, exercise can also stimulate the production of oxidative free radicals, but physical activity also enhances your body's antioxidant enzymes systems that get rid of them naturally and may help prevent diabetes complications for that reason.

Key Behaviors to Prevent Health Complications
- Focus on losing at least 5-7 percent of your body weight and maintain that new, lower body weight over time.
- Regularly monitor your blood glucose levels and make adjustments to control them.

continued

- Make healthier food choices by eating fewer refined and highly processed foods and more of those that are naturally rich in antioxidants, vitamins, minerals and fiber.
- Exercise and stay as physically active as possible on a daily basis, especially when you're dieting, so you'll retain more of your muscle mass.
- Find a knowledgable doctor, preferably an endocrinologist if you have type 1 diabetes, or a diabetes educator that you trust who can help you better manage your condition.
- Always take your prescribed oral medications, insulin or other injectable diabetes medications to control your blood glucose.
- Set SMART goals focusing on maintenance of your good health habits.
- Involve a supportive spouse, family or friends in your weight loss habits and managing your diabetes.
- Maintain a positive attitude about your body weight, diabetes and life in general.

WHY FITNESS MATTERS (AND HOW TO GET MORE FIT)

In recent weeks, you started to get a better feel for how resistance training can help you reach your weight goals, but now you'll additionally be focusing on beefing up your aerobic training. Adding in interval training can boost how much blood glucose your muscles use up, and how fit you get, which is critically important when it comes to living long and well (with or without diabetes). The interval training that the Diabetes Breakthrough program includes as part of its exercise program is easy to do and beneficial to your fitness level and blood glucose control.

PLAN WORKOUTS AND VARY THEM FOR BEST RESULTS

There really is a lot of flexibility when it comes to what you do to get more physically active. However, to get the most out of any activity that you do, you should consider adding in intervals of any length that cause you to work harder for short periods of time. You may think you're doing enough walking already, but now is the time to learn to get the greatest blood glucose and weight loss benefits from your activities.

You can also get more fit in less time (and lower your blood glucose more) by adding some harder intervals into any aerobic activity that you're doing. That may just mean picking one of the interval profiles on fitness training machines or walking faster between two mailboxes from time to time when you're out for your daily walk. The options for integrating interval training into your workouts are endless and the benefits to your health are almost limitless.

Benefits of Interval Training

- Burns more total fat and glucose (calories) than steady pace aerobic training.
- Improves diabetes control.
- Builds endurance and speed.
- Strengthens your heart muscle.
- Goes faster and is less boring.
- Extends calorie-burning of muscles and body beyond the exercise session.

YOUR EXERCISE PLAN FOR WEEK 5

This week you'll be adding some interval training to rev up your workouts. It's nothing to be fearful of. Just plan on trying to add in some faster intervals into any workouts you're already doing, starting with one to two days per week and progressing to three or more. The intervals can vary in length from as little as 10 seconds to up to a minute or more and you can add them in as often as you like. We recommend that you start with 20 second faster sprints, separated by one minute and 40 seconds of a slower intensity to recover. Circuit training itself is already a lot like interval training, so try doing it in place of one of your more basic aerobic training days.

WEEK 5: DIABETES BREAKTHROUGH EXERCISE PLAN

DAY	AEROBIC	RESISTANCE	STRETCHING	TYPES OF EXERCISE
1	12 minutes	25 minutes	3 minutes	Aerobic, including interval training (20-second sprints, 1 minute and 40 seconds of recovery)
2	37 minutes		3 minutes	
3	12 minutes	25 minutes	3 minutes	Resistance (3 sets, 15 repetitions)
4				Stretching
5	12 minutes	25 minutes	3 minutes	
6	37 minutes		3 minutes	
7				

TOTAL TIME: 40 MINUTES

The trick is to make interval training specific to your aerobic activities. First, spend three to five minutes warming up at an easy pace. Once you're warmed up, start the main part of your workout, but make sure to watch the clock and change your speed or intensity based on your chosen interval time. Your heart rate and breathing will be further elevated during the interval segment. Follow this with a recovery segment performed at a lower intensity based on the time allocated.

Examples of Interval Training

Walking intervals: Start with 3–5 minutes of a warm-up at low intensity. Speed up to 3.0 miles per hour (mph) for 1 minute. Increase your speed to 3.5 mph or increase the incline (if you're on your treadmill) to 3 percent for 20 seconds and then reduce your speed back to 3.0 mph for 1 minute and 40 seconds. Repeat the intervals as frequently as you can for best results (and vary their intensity, too). You should try to complete 20 minutes of intervals at a time.

Bicycling intervals: Start with 3-5 minutes of a warm-up at a lower cycling intensity. Choose a level (resistance) that you can maintain, such as 60 revolutions per minute (rpm). For the interval portion, stay at the same level, but increase to at least 90 rpm, or stay at 60 rpm and increase the level by 2-3 grades (e.g., level 4 up to level 6 or 7). Alternate 20-second intervals with 1 minute and 40 seconds of recovery for 20 minutes or more. Since interval training requires a significant amount of energy, you can perform it when you are short on time since even 20 or 30 minutes will usually suffice.

HOW TO MANAGE DIABETES ON SICK DAYS

What happens to your blood glucose levels on sick days? One of the reasons that you may have hyperglycemia on those days is that you are sick or have an infection of some sort. Any type of physical stress like that on the body can cause elevations in hormones that raise your blood glucose levels. So, on sick days, you'll need to pay extra attention to your self-care to control your blood glucose levels. A "sick day" is one when you may be experiencing:

- An illness (e.g., cold, flu)
- An infection
- Nausea, vomiting or diarrhea
- An injury or surgery
- Dental problems or any kind of major stress

Being sick affects how your body uses glucose. Sick days can cause high blood glucose because your body needs more energy to deal with the physical stress of illness. More glucose is released from your liver to provide the extra energy you need to recover and levels of your stress hormones also increase. In fact, your blood glucose may increase to a higher level than is healthy for your body and can impair your ability to get well or to overcome an infection.

When you are sick you need to check your blood glucose more often, drink more water and other calorie-free fluids and possibly adjust your medications, particularly if you have two or more blood glucose readings within 24 hours that are above 250 mg/dl. It's a good practice to check your blood glucose four times a day for a mild illness (e.g., cold, flu or gastrointestinal virus) and every three to four hours for more severe illness. Also check more often if you are having a procedure like dental work or a colonoscopy done. Be sure to get plenty of rest and avoid physical activity.

On sick days, it's extra important to stay well hydrated. High blood glucose may cause you to urinate more, resulting in dehydration. Drink eight ounces of sugar-free fluids every one to two hours. If you feel too sick to eat, switch back and forth between drinks that contain sugar and drinks without any so that your blood glucose levels don't get too high or too low. However, if you can eat, try to maintain your Diabetes Breakthrough meal plan while drinking plenty of sugar-free beverages.

Certain situations and signs necessitate a call for help, including being unable to keep down fluids, blood glucose levels over 250 mg/dl, persistent stomach pains, vomiting, diarrhea or fever above 101 degrees. Immediately report unusually high glucose readings to your health care provider, especially if you can't keep food, medications or fluids down.

IT'S NOT JUST SIZE THAT MATTERS

For LaTasha, what happened to her was the Joslin Why WAIT program. "I think that this program has really turned my life around," she says. "It changed how I view weight loss. Before it was always just about the size of my jeans. It was really never about what was going on inside and how my weight was affecting my body and my life." The more she learned about how her lifestyle choices affect her body not only now, but also in the near future, the more she realized that the choice to live or not live a healthy life was up to her.

Now she is exercising regularly and never uses an excuse to get out of doing it. "It's really something when I'm working out and I'm thinking figuratively about how I'm opening the door and getting the glucose into the cells instead of things that are less important . . . like what size I'm wearing." But she's wearing smaller jeans now and she has more energy than she ever remembers having before. "The program totally changed the way I think about everything . . . and I never want to go back to my old way of thinking." With a new attitude like that, she probably never will.

DIABETES BREAKTHROUGH WEEK 6

Diets and Dieting, Core Training, Yoga and Changing Your Negative Thoughts

Confused by all the diets out there? So are we. Low-carbohydrate, no-carbohydrate, low-fat, single food diets . . . the list goes on and on. Many of the bestselling nonfiction books these days are also diet books and yet everyone keeps getting heavier. This week we'll discuss the good and the bad about diets and what makes this program's meal plan and other activities so different from the rest.

With healthy eating in mind, you'll practice making a balanced salad for lunch or dinner that is tasty and good for weight loss. You'll start working on strengthening your body core with targeted exercises that will make you stronger. You will also learn some yoga poses that benefit your strength and flexibility and have a calming effect that helps you better manage your blood glucose levels. Finally, you'll explore how your destructive thoughts can undermine your weight loss goals and what to do to change your thought patterns for the better.

CONFESSIONS OF A PROFESSIONAL DIETER

Elaine was a diet pro: she'd been on every commercial program known to mankind over the past 25 years. Like most chronic dieters, her problem wasn't losing weight—she could do that just fine. Rather, it was keeping it off afterward. How would you guess she did on and following the Joslin Why WAIT program? We'll tell you later.

WHY ALL DIETS ARE NOT EQUAL

While it's possible to lose weight on any type of diet that cuts calories, the truth is that all diets are not equal when it comes to maintaining your new, lower body weight. Severely restrictive ones, like the Atkins low-carbohydrate plan, are nearly impossible to sustain over a lifetime and it's very common after finishing that diet and other popular ones to gain all the weight back. What's more, high-fat diets that emphasize animal fats like bacon, butter and sour cream are just not that healthy for your heart once you stop losing weight. However, simply picking foods that cause less of a blood glucose spike after eating helps people with diabetes lose weight, according to a study in the *Journal of Nutrition.*

TEST WHAT YOU KNOW ABOUT DIETING

You may think that going on another diet is the answer to your weight problem, but, as you may already know, it's really easy to gain back the weight you've lost . . . and then some. This yo-yo dieting can make you less healthy in the long run because you may lose both fat and muscle, but only gain fat back—leaving you with more body fat than when you started.

Find out what you know about dieting and fad diets with this short quiz:

1. **Which of these fad diets is likely to make you lose the most weight overall?**
    a. Shangri-La Diet
    b. Fruit Flush Diet
    c. French Women Don't Get Fat Plan
    d. Cabbage Soup Diet
    e. Morning Banana Diet
    f. All of these diets would work—as long as you take in fewer calories than you need (but they're definitely not all equally healthy for you)

2.   **Which of the following diets is healthiest for you with diabetes when you're trying to control your blood glucose?**
     a. Mediterranean Diet
     b. DASH Diet
     c. Zone Diet
     d. Glycemic Index Diet
     e. Joslin Why WAIT Diet
     f. All of these diets are healthy and would help manage blood glucose

3.   **When you're dieting to lose weight, what is the best way to guarantee that you're losing the bad "visceral" fat from inside your belly?**
     a. Eat fewer calories every day
     b. Burn extra calories with exercise
     c. Eat fewer calories and do aerobic exercise
     d. Eat fewer calories and do resistance training
     e. Eat fewer calories and do any type of exercise
     f. All of these except for "eat fewer calories every day" without exercising

P.S. The answers to the quiz are: (1) f (it's the lack of calories that causes weight loss, not the intake of certain types of food); (2) f (all of these are healthy diets that help you manage blood glucose and body weight; however, the Joslin Why WAIT Diet has been proven to help you maintain long-term weight loss); and (3) f (any type of exercise can help get rid of deep belly fat, but dieting alone can't).

THE KEYS ARE MORE PROTEIN AND A BALANCED DIET

The popularity of low-carbohydrate diets including Atkins and South Beach may have led you to think that all carbohydrates are bad and cause weight gain when, in fact, whole grains, beans, fruits, vegetables and other carb-based foods do just the opposite by delivering essential vitamins and minerals, fiber and a host of important phytonutrients to your body. Based on the research, you shouldn't lower your total carbohydrate intake to fewer than 130 grams a day, which is why the Joslin Why WAIT program developed a balance with 40–45 percent of total calories coming from carbohydrates. This percentage is lower than what most people eat, but it's high enough to avoid the bad health consequences caused by low-carbohydrate diets.

The bottom line, however, is that you can't lose weight or reverse your diabetes without taking in fewer calories while changing your dietary composition. Another key to the Joslin Why WAIT program's dietary success is its emphasis on the amount and quality of protein, carbohydrate and fat. The latest research shows that if you even just moderately increase your daily protein intake (to 20–30 percent of calories), it helps manage blood glucose, promote weight loss and improve your blood pressure, cholesterol levels and other health markers. Increasing your protein intake to 1–1.5 grams per kilogram of body weight (or about 20–30 percent of total calories) when you cut back on your total calorie intake works well for anyone who needs to lose weight and has type 2 diabetes. Eating more protein also makes you less hungry, fills you up faster, burns more daily calories and—probably most important of all—keeps you from losing muscle when you're dieting and exercising regularly.

On top of that, cutting your carbohydrates down to 40–45 percent of your daily calories helps you lose more visceral fat and increases your good cholesterol (HDL). Since you also get to take in about 30–35 percent of your calories as fat, you don't have to avoid nuts, avocados, olives and other healthy types of fat. That's how this program allows you to improve your health while watching your excess pounds melt away.

CREATE A NUTRIENT BALANCED SALAD

Visualizing a plate of food with a carbohydrate food fitting on one-third of it can help you plan meals well. Let's do an exercise with a salad as an example that will help you see how all of this information about portion size works in real life with all of your meal choices. This way you can start to piece together various meals when you're eating out as well as at home.

In this case, your mission is to create a balanced salad with our recommended percentages of macronutrients. What would you include in your salad? What would provide your protein (20–30 percent of calories), carbohydrate (40–45 percent) and fat (30–35 percent)? How would you determine the portions?

Vegetables-Carbs-Protein/Fat Plate

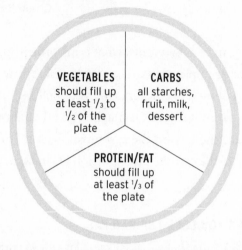

VEGETABLES
should fill up
at least $\frac{1}{3}$ to
$\frac{1}{2}$ of the
plate

CARBS
all starches,
fruit, milk,
dessert

PROTEIN/FAT
should fill up
at least $\frac{1}{3}$ of
the plate

A list of the ingredients you have available to use follows. Let's look at the vegetables. Are the vegetables "free"? Yes, they all actually are. What about some carbohydrate options for your salad? One thing to know is that carbohydrates always trump everything else, so even if the food is comprised of both carbohydrate and protein, it should be counted on your plate as only carbohydrate. For instance, hummus, even though it is a protein, should be counted as a carb because it is made from chickpeas, which are primarily carbohydrate-based.

Vegetable Choices	Protein/Fat Choices	Carbohydrate Choices
• Lettuce	• Chicken	• Potato salad
• Tomatoes	• Egg	• Black beans
• Shredded carrots	• Feta cheese	• Pasta salad
• Green peppers	• Shredded cheese	• Chickpeas/hummus
• Broccoli	• Cottage cheese	• Dried cranberries

continued

Vegetable Choices	Protein/Fat Choices	Carbohydrate Choices
• Cauliflower	• Olives	• Mandarin oranges
• Cucumber	• Sunflower seeds	• Melon
• Onion	• Dressing	• Peas
• Celery	• Oil/Vinegar	• Beets
• Vinegar only		• Croutons

Ask yourself, "What is my carbohydrate, what is my protein and fat and what is my vegetable?" For example, think to yourself, "Here's my salad, starting with lettuce. All I've got on it is chicken, a hard-boiled egg and some dressing. I'm missing the carbohydrate." Or maybe your thought is, "All I've got is pasta salad so I have the fat and the carbohydrate, but I'm missing some protein." Just make sure the carbohydrate portion fits in no more than a third of your plate.

WHY EXERCISE HELPS YOU LOSE THE BAD FAT

We've known for a long time that storing excess fat within your belly (known as visceral fat) is bad for your health. If you have a lot, it increases your risk for heart disease, high blood pressure and even type 2 diabetes.

We also know that both aerobic and resistance training are more effective at helping you lose visceral fat than dieting is. New research published in *Obesity* examined how improving lifestyle habits helped men diagnosed with obesity with too much belly fat. While exercise helped them burn more bad fat, having a healthier diet also kept their insulin working better, showing that it's beneficial to make both changes at once. What's more, another study showed that doing interval training while cutting back on carbohydrates and eating fewer calories for 14 days ensures that you lose bad fat while keeping more muscle.

The Diabetes Breakthrough program is designed to help you retain your muscle mass and possibly gain more through resistance training that will boost your metabolism, lower your blood glucose and prevent you from gaining weight back. With the design of this program, you'll also maximize your loss of bad belly fat.

YOUR EXERCISE PLAN FOR WEEK 6

This week you'll learn about core stability training, exercises that work your core muscles (i.e., abdomen and lower back), which you can do on one or two days this week. You'll also get to try out some yoga poses as part of your usual stretching routine. Yoga can also double as part of your resistance training when it comes to improving your muscular endurance and not just strength one or more days this week. Keep mixing up your exercise for the best results and to keep from getting bored with your routine.

WEEK 6: DIABETES BREAKTHROUGH EXERCISE PLAN

DAY	AEROBIC	RESISTANCE	STRETCHING	TYPES OF EXERCISE
1	16 minutes	25 minutes	4 minutes	Aerobic, including interval training
2	41 minutes		4 minutes	(20-second sprints, 1 minute and 40 seconds of recovery)
3	16 minutes	25 minutes	4 minutes	Resistance (3 sets, 15 repetitions)
4				Core stability
5	16 minutes	25 minutes	4 minutes	Yoga
6	41 minutes		4 minutes	Stretching
7				

TOTAL TIME: 45 MINUTES

WHAT IS CORE STABILITY TRAINING?

Core stability training is a series of exercises aimed at developing strength in abdominal and lower back areas, or the "core" of the body. Your core strength allows your body to stabilize itself during all types of movement. Thus, inner strength allows for the flow of strength to the rest of the body.

Benefits of Core Training

- Reduces risk of injury during exercise and daily activities.
- Provides a strong base of support for all movements.
- Supports the spine and improves posture.
- Prevents or reduces low-back pain.
- Creates strength and stabilizes the trunk of your body.
- Enables you to perform exercises and movements in a better coordinated and stronger manner, especially those that involve both upper and lower body activities.
- Tightens and shapes muscles in the core area, which may reduce waist size.
- Helps with developing better balance and coordination.

CORE STABILITY EXERCISES

Try these easy exercises to build a stronger core. If you don't have an exercise ball, you can modify the exercises that use it by using a large pillow or similar item to support your back.

1. **ABDOMINALS—Crunch**

   Place your arms across
   your upper chest. For added
   resistance, hold a dumbbell
   on your upper chest with your
   lower back supported. Tighten
   your abdominals by bringing
   your ribs toward your pelvis
   until your shoulders clear the
   exercise ball and breathe out.
   Return to the starting position
   while breathing in.

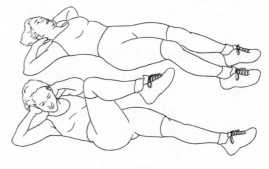

2. **ABDOMINALS—Crunches
   (Scissor Kick/Twist)**

   Tighten your abdominals,
   raise your upper body
   and twist to the side. Your
   elbow does not need to
   actually touch your opposite
   (raised) knee. Alternate
   sides and breathe in and out
   throughout this exercise.

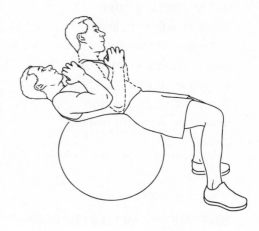

3. **TRUNK STABILITY—Bridging**

   Slowly raise your buttocks
   from the floor, keeping your
   stomach tight. Gently lower
   your back to the ground
   and repeat. Breathe in and
   out throughout this exercise.

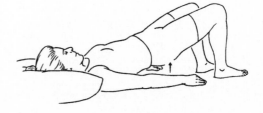

4. TRUNK STABILITY—Bridging with Straight Leg Raise

With your legs bent, lift your buttocks up off the floor. Then slowly extend your left knee, keeping your stomach tight. Repeat with the other leg. Breathe in and out throughout this exercise.

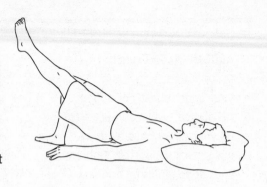

5. CORE STABILITY AND LEG STRENGTH— Leg Extension (Ball)

While sitting on an exercise ball, place hands on your thighs or hold them up and bent at the elbow if you have dumbbells. Extend leg at one knee and hold for two to five seconds while engaging your core muscles to hold your body still in the position. Return back to starting position and extend other knee. If no exercise ball is available, do this exercise sitting on the edge of a chair or sofa. If holding dumbbells, straighten arms at the elbows to increase difficulty during this exercise.

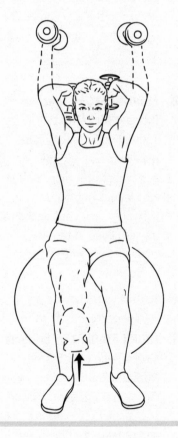

6. CORE STABILITY—Plank and Modified Plank

Bend your elbows 90 degrees and rest your weight on your forearms. Your elbows should be directly beneath your shoulders and your body should form a straight line from your head to your feet. Hold the position 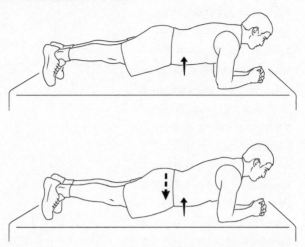 for as long as you can and repeat. If this exercise is too hard when you start doing it, do a modified plank by bending your knees and resting on them instead. If you have shoulder or elbow problems, you may need to avoid this exercise. If your eye doctor told you that you have diabetic retinopathy or bleeding in eyes, you should avoid this exercise to prevent extra pressure in the retina.

7. BACK—Lumbar Rotation Stretch

Lie on your back with your left knee drawn toward your chest. Slowly bring your bent leg across your body 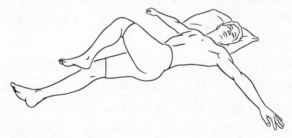 until you feel the stretch in your lower back/hip area. Hold and repeat on the other side.

8. TRUNK—Twist (Standing)

With your resistance band anchored at chest height and your side toward it with a wide stance, keep your thumbs up as you pull away from the anchor while squeezing your abs and breathing out. Keep your arm that is farthest from the anchor straight. Return to your starting position in a slow controlled motion while breathing in. Face the other way and repeat on the other side.

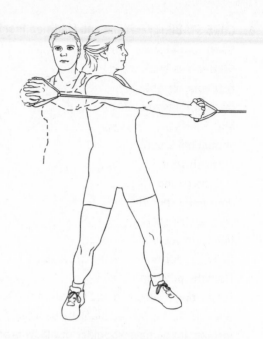

YOGA POSES

Yoga means "union" in Sanskrit, the language of ancient India where this exercise originated. It denotes the connection between mind, body and spirit through the practice of physical poses while concentrating on breathing and being in the moment.

Learning yoga poses and practicing regularly gives you the chance to build strength and flexibility simultaneously, helps you become more aware of your posture and gets you to focus on the moment. In general, standing poses are the foundation of many other more complex ones in yoga, making them an ideal place to start. Concentrate on aligning your full body and maintaining balance while you breathe in and out slowly and fully during each pose. Start by holding a position for two breaths. As you get stronger, increase to four or five breaths.

1. YOGA—Mountain Pose (Tadasana)

Stand as tall as possible, with your feet together and your arms straight down by your sides. Make all quadrants of your feet touch the floor evenly, expand your ribs, straighten your spine, hold your head straight on top and fully extend your hands and fingers. Hold for five breaths. Inhale and exhale through your nose. If it is difficult for you, you may inhale through your nose and exhale through your mouth.

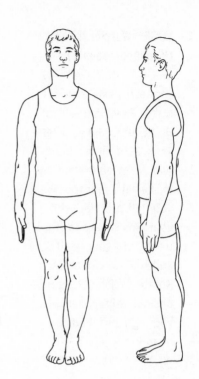

2. YOGA—Warrior I Pose (Virabhadrasana I)

Standing in a wide stride, rotate your back leg out 20 degrees to ground your foot and stretch your hands up to the sky. Bend your front leg 90 degrees and look up while reaching up over your head. Hold for two breaths and repeat with your other leg forward.

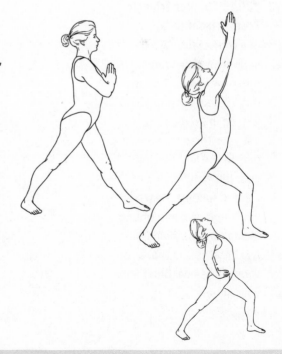

3. YOGA—Warrior II Pose (Virabhadrasana II)

In a wide stance with your arms extended out, rotate your right leg out 90 degrees and your left leg in 20 degrees. Bend your right leg 90 degrees in line with your foot. Keep your left foot flat, with your hips square to your front. Turn your head right and hold for two breaths. Rotate back to a center position and repeat with your feet switched and head to the left.

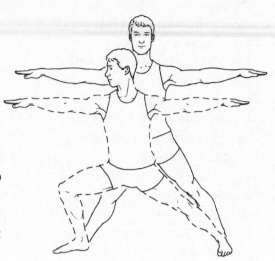

4. YOGA—Counter Triangle Pose (Trikonasana)

In a wide stance with your arms extended out, rotate your right leg out 90 degrees and your left leg in 20 degrees. Tilt your torso from your hips to the left, placing your left hand on your calf for support. Reach your right arm straight up facing upward. Hold for two breaths and repeat on your other side. Don't lock your knees.

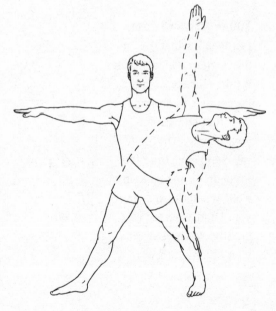

5. YOGA—Long Angle Pose (Parsvakonasana)

In a wide stance with your arms extended out, rotate your right leg out 90 degrees and your left leg in 20 degrees. Bend your right leg 90 degrees and tilt your torso from your hips over your right leg. Place your right forearm on your right thigh if you are a beginner to support your body. Extend your left arm upward. Keep your focus forward and hold for two breaths before repeating on the other side. Don't lock your knees.

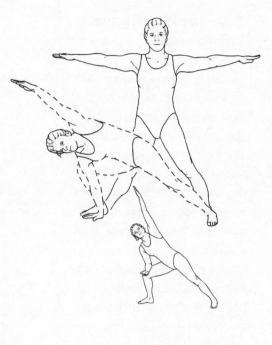

6. YOGA—Chair Pose (Utkatasana)

With your feet together, bend your knees 90 degrees, keeping your back straight. Reach your arms over your head, sitting your hips back toward your heels. Keep your focus straight and hold for two breaths.

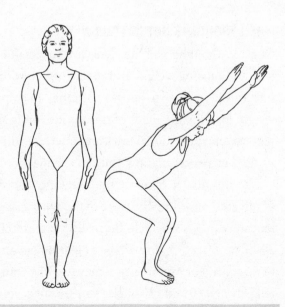

7. YOGA—Tree Pose (Vrksasana)

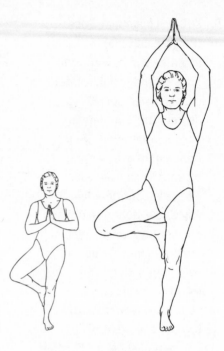

With your weight distributed equally on all four corners of both feet and your hands in a prayer position in front of you, bend your right knee, bringing the sole of your right foot high onto your inner left thigh. Keep both of your hips squared toward the front. Focus on something that doesn't move to help you keep your balance. Repeat the move while standing on your right foot. If you cannot bring your right foot high inside your left thigh when you first try this pose, bring it lower onto your left leg, but avoid placing your foot directly on the inside of your knee.

WHEN THOUGHTS GET IN YOUR WAY

Negative thoughts can interfere with successful behavior change of any kind, including losing weight and managing your diabetes. But recognizing and interrupting negative thought patterns can help you stick with your plans for weight loss. So, the focus of this discussion is about which negative thought patterns can pull you off track and interfere with your efforts to improve your health behaviors and how you can change them.

We are going to focus on the "thinking" aspect because there has been a lot of research regarding the types of thoughts that derail people trying to change longstanding habits, including eating and exercise habits. Black-and-white or all-or-nothing thinking can be a big problem and it's easy to get into that type of mindset. For example, you may feel like your blood glucose levels need to fall between 80 and 130 or else you are not accomplishing anything. You don't want bad news, so you may choose to completely stop using your meter. The problem is that the minute you put that meter away, you have forsaken your most useful diabetes tool.

Of course, there are textbook goals of having blood glucose readings between 80 and 130 or an A1C below 6.5 or 7 percent, but these are ideal goals to work toward, not a standard with which to criticize yourself or to minimize your progress. You need to think about what these goals mean for you as an individual and how you can make them work for you over the course of your entire life rather than just over a short period of time. Keep your eye on your long-term goals, not just your more immediate ones.

STOP NEGATIVE THINKING ABOUT YOUR WEIGHT

This same kind of black-and-white or all-or-nothing thinking might get triggered if you weigh yourself and see either no change or an increase in the number on the scale. People can be very vulnerable to slipping into negative thinking in this situation, telling themselves things like, "Nothing I do matters" or "All my hard work hasn't amounted to anything." These statements are simply untrue.

It's important to come up with ways to challenge automatic negative thoughts. Your weight loss may not be consistent from one week to another and lead to negative thinking about your progress. Stepping back and seeing the overall downward trend is important so that you see that you really are achieving your overall goal.

This task of losing weight and improving diabetes control can feel overwhelming. For example, you can make changes and not see any improvements in your weight loss some weeks. Remember, however, that there can be a cascade effect, meaning that it's possible for your weight to be stable or even go up a little at first while your blood glucose is going down. Not everything works in exact parallel: sometimes blood glucose can improve more quickly than weight can, or maybe some other health marker that you aren't measuring is what has improved that week. Your individual weight loss will likely vary and you should only look for your own unique patterns so that you aren't discouraged by weeks during which things don't go as well as you would like them to (either with regard to losing weight or managing diabetes).

THE HIGHWAY, NOT MY WAY

The Diabetes Breakthrough program uses a highway metaphor to represent forward progress on different highways—the blood glucose highway and the weight management highway (and actually multiple other highways including fitness level, energy/mood, cardiac risk factors like cholesterol and blood pressure, etc.). As you are changing your health behaviors, it's as if you are driving down multiple lanes in the highway all at the same time, but traffic in each lane may be traveling at different speeds. Encountering a roadblock on the blood glucose highway can lead to negative thoughts, which may discourage you from checking your blood glucose and working to keep it within target range—and the same can be true for your weight.

A detour from the weight loss highway could bring you into a similar cycle of negative thinking. For example, you may be tempted to say to yourself, "I thought I would lose a certain amount of weight each week, but this week I lost less than I expected. This isn't working and it never will. I give up." This type of negative thinking can come up any time you're trying to change a behavior. You may need to constantly rework your thoughts and plans to get back on the highway.

If you think about it, when you get off at the wrong exit or take a detour when you are driving in real life, you may get frustrated and annoyed, but you rarely beat yourself up in the same way you do when you make an eating, blood glucose or exercise slip. When lost in real life, you get into problem-solving mode and try to figure out how to get back to the highway. You don't start investing in real estate in the town where you got lost or get a library card there. You have to start applying problem-solving strategies to health-related slips, or you will stay off at the wrong exit long-term. Think of some of the skills you are learning in this program as a road map for this multiple-lane health highway.

In the next section, you will see some negative thoughts listed. Do any of these look familiar? What are the different types of negative thinking you notice that you have fallen into in the past when you try to lose weight and improve your diabetes control? You will likely find some items that look very familiar and others that don't really fit your particular thinking style. The idea is to identify which types of thoughts are most likely to happen to you and then learn to respond to those thoughts differently.

If you have trouble challenging these thoughts on your own, focus on the four questions (that follow). These questions are a simple tool to help you challenge your negative thinking and continue to move along the path of ongoing behavior change. It's not realistic to expect that you will never have another negative thought again, it happens to all of us. The important thing is to stay alert to negative thoughts when they arise and use "talking back" or these questions to get yourself back on track. You don't have to stay stuck in negative thinking.

Four Questions to Ask Yourself

When you recognize yourself engaging in "roadblock thinking," try asking yourself these questions:

1. Does this thought help me reach my goal or create a barrier to my health?
2. Where did I learn this thought?
3. Is this thought logical?
4. Is this thought true?

Adapted from *Self-Nurture* by Alice Domar, Ph.D. (Penguin Books, 2001).

PRACTICE CHANGING YOUR AUTOMATIC NEGATIVE THINKING

A number of different types of negative thinking are included in this section, along with some examples. Take a few minutes to·think through how you might change these ways of thinking for yourself.

Black-and-White/All-or-Nothing Thinking

Example: "I'm either on the plan or I've cheated and failed." If you don't stick to exercise, meal plan or weight loss perfectly, you feel like you are failing.

Try talking back with: "I am working at making changes gradually." "What can I learn from this and try to do differently next time?"

Write down your own negative thoughts and ways to challenge them here:

_____

_____

_____

_____

Mental Filter or Disqualifying the Positive

You pick out a single negative detail and dwell on that until the whole picture looks bad. You discount real, positive changes by focusing exclusively on the negative.

Examples: "What good is losing only five pounds when I have 25 to go?" "So what if I've cut my medications? I still have diabetes."

Try talking back with: "I need to focus on what I've already learned and accomplished and build from there."

Add your own talking back points here:

_____

_____

_____

_____

Not Acknowledging Your Hard Work

Example: "The only reason this is working is because of the meal replacement shakes."

Try talking back with: "I can prove that I can do this on my own by starting to add in some meals in place of the shakes."

Add your own talking back points here:

_____

_____

_____

_____

"Should" Statements or Moral Judgments

Examples: "I should be able to just do it." "I don't have any willpower."

Try talking back with: "This is a process. Criticizing and blaming myself does not help."

Add your own talking back points here:

_____

_____

_____

_____

Rationalization

Blaming others or a situation outside yourself for problems you may be having with maintaining progress is a rationalization.

Examples: "I can't exercise in this weather." "I can't say no when my mother offers me seconds."

Try talking back with: "How I respond to these barriers is up to me. It's my choice."

Add your own talking back points here:

_____

_____

_____

_____

Not As Good As Thoughts

The risk of having friends, family, colleagues and others around you is that you may find it hard not to compare yourself with the progress of others.

Example: "Someone else always seems to lose way more weight than I have ... and it seems like she doesn't even have to work at it."

Try talking back with: "Every one of us is going to have our own successes and problems."

Add your own talking back points here:

_____

_____

_____

_____

Giving Up

Examples: "I've heard all this before." "I've tried all this before and it never helped."

Try talking back with: "I need to focus on one step at a time." "My health and life are worth this effort."

Add your own talking back points here:

_____

_____

_____

_____

A DIET PRO NO LONGER

Remember our diet professional, Elaine? Her experiences with the Joslin Why WAIT program were notably different from any of the other diets she tried over a quarter of a century. She was also the queen of negative thinking.

But for her, this program was finally different from all the failed ones in her past. "While most of these other weight loss programs have some excellent features, none of them helped me lose weight as quickly and as easily as the Why WAIT program," she says with enthusiasm. "It's the combination of things that really worked for me this time. The diet plan really kept me from being hungry and the exercise was fun because it was different every day. I also learned a lot about controlling negative thinking and that helped me, too. I lost almost 40 pounds in record time and have kept most of it off for over a year."

DIABETES BREAKTHROUGH WEEK 7

Social Eating, Superset Training and Becoming an Active Exerciser

---

This week is all about others—namely engaging with other people and using social connections to help you reach your goals, while trying out some other forms of physical activity. Super Bowl party coming up? Wedding to go to? You will also find out more about how to survive social eating situations and you'll be introduced to "superset" training that gives you a great workout when your time is limited. This week you will learn about recognizing and overcoming your barriers to becoming an active exerciser.

USE YOUR SOCIAL CONNECTIONS

Claudia is undeniably a people person who really doesn't like doing things such as exercising on her own. Enter the Joslin Why WAIT program. "We all enrolled in the program with substantial health issues and more to follow if we did not come to grips with our weight," she recalls. "What really worked for me is that we were able to form a group where we felt comfortable enough with each other to share successes as well as slips, to discuss how our program was impacting our families and how we were adjusting psychologically to our new selves." Give some thought to what you think would work for you.

YOU ARE WHAT YOUR FRIENDS EAT

By this week, you've learned why it's important to set SMART goals, monitor your blood glucose and more. In weeks to come, you'll be focusing on controlling your cravings and managing your stress levels, too. Doing all of these things will help you to finally overcome your inability to lose weight and keep it off—which is not about a simple lack of willpower or motivation, but rather about behaviors that you can learn to manage.

What you may not have realized yet is how much you're influenced by others in your social networks. Do you find yourself snacking when you're not hungry, bingeing on pizza or having another beer when you don't really want one? Research published in the *American Journal of Public Health* suggests that eating patterns are often shared among friends and family members, especially spouses. What you snack on and how much you drink is affected by spouses, friends and siblings. Holding back especially when everyone around you is indulging can lead you to start obsessing about your food and having strong cravings. You may or may not act on those urges right away, but if you ever get depressed, you're more likely to (and depression is a common affliction in people with diabetes). This is all the more reason to find ways to make your lifestyle changes a habit.

Have you ever considered that to lose weight and change your lifestyle, you may have to get your family and friends involved, as well? Bring them along for the ride while you change your eating and exercise patterns for the better. Their health can benefit along with yours and you will have all the social support that you need to continue with your healthier lifestyle once you finish the Diabetes Breakthrough program.

If you've been feeling down from time to time, keep in mind that depression can also cause you to give in to your cravings and lead you to binge on foods that you would otherwise be able to resist. Both healthier eating and regular physical activity can help you manage your depressive symptoms, anxiety and stress levels.

Speaking of Eating: Shake Less, Eat More

If you have been using meal replacement shakes in place of breakfast and/or lunch, this week you should start transitioning over to following suggested menus for a healthy breakfast and lunch instead. The goal is to return to "normal" eating as much as possible (while still keeping your calories reduced) to allow you to experience more real-world eating like you'll be doing for the rest of your life when this program ends. By way of reminder, you'll find healthy breakfast choices and sample menus in Appendix A and lunch suggestions, menus and recipes in Appendix B.

BE SUCCESSFUL AT SOCIAL EATING

Three primary skills can be used to navigate social eating and maintain healthy choices: preplanning, sticking to those plans and assertive communication. This week, we'll be talking about these strategies so you can use them when eating socially at restaurants, meetings or parties. These can be challenging situations when you're working on controlling both your weight and your diabetes.

What are some of the problems you've faced in social settings like parties or meetings or eating out with friends? One of the themes throughout the Diabetes Breakthrough program has been the importance of planning—planning what and when you'll eat and when and how often you'll exercise, monitor your blood glucose and take your medications. Good planning applies here, as well. This is a great time to use the SMART goals approach.

Can you think of an example of a SMART goal around social eating? By coming up with such goals in advance, you'll be more likely to stick with your plan. Saying "I just won't eat much at the party" isn't as effective as "I will take two servings of the healthy food that I am bringing to the party, along with unlimited veggies and I will sit as far from the food table as I can." As another example for restaurants, rather than saying you "just won't eat the bread," you can ask the waiter to remove the bread basket from the table.

Having a social eating strategy and adhering to the plan are essential skills to practice. Think about some of the things that are working for you with regard to planning ahead and sticking to those plans. Use those whenever possible.

Let's talk about the final skill, assertive communication, which is asking for what you want in an effective way. We're sure you've been in situations where you've asked directly for what you want, such as having salad dressing served on the side to reduce the calorie content of a meal. Not everyone is comfortable asking for what they want, however. Sometimes people feel awkward or rude making special requests. It may just take some practice, but you can communicate your needs firmly without being rude.

TAKE THESE STEPS

You can take these steps to change your life for the better when eating in social situations. The more you practice doing them, the easier they will become.

Step One: Plan ahead, plan ahead, plan ahead, plan ahead

The most important step in learning to handle social eating successfully is to plan ahead. The more you can plan ahead, the more likely you are to stay within your meal plan goals *and* not feel deprived or guilty.

Things to try:
- Call ahead to a restaurant or check its menu online so you can plan what to order ahead of time, or choose another restaurant with healthier food choices.
- By anticipating a restaurant meal, a small amount of calories can be "banked" ahead. Be careful doing this, though, as overly restrictive eating can change your metabolism and/or set you up to overeat in response to hunger. Don't completely skip any meals in anticipation of eating out later on.
- Order first and don't linger over the menu choices; your goal is to increase your chances of sticking to a healthier choice. Keep in mind that menus are designed to make everything sound irresistible.
- Don't drink more than the recommended daily amounts of alcohol (one drink for women, two for men). Generally, alcohol

just adds empty calories with little nutritional value and those coming from the very occasional glass of wine or other drink must be factored into your meal plan.

- If you are eating at someone else's home, ask the host of a party or dinner what he/she plans on serving and offer to bring something that ensures you'll have at least one healthy food choice.
- Mingle and socialize to help keep away from buffet tables and snacks. Try focusing on the noneating aspects of the event.

Step Two: Ask for what you want and need

Sometimes people feel awkward or rude making special requests in restaurants or at dinner parties. It takes practice in order to feel comfortable making special requests.

Techniques for sounding assertive, but not rude:
- Begin with "I" not "You."
- Using "I" statements shows that you're taking responsibility for your own feelings and desires. Using "you" often puts others on the defensive.
- *"You" statement:* "You didn't put the salad dressing on the side."
- *"I" statement:* "I asked to have the salad dressing on the side, please."
- Always start with: "I would like . . ." "I need . . ." or "I will have. . . ."
- Use a firm and friendly tone of voice, combined with a smile.
- Look the person you're speaking with in the eye.
- Repeat your needs until they are heard and understood. Sometimes it may take several tries.

SPECIAL ORDERS ARE YOUR RIGHT

When eating out, it's your right to make healthy food choices and eat smaller portions. You can be in control of your meal. Make substitutions or get things on the side. If you are willing to be assertive, you can really improve many menu items.

Here are some great tips for ordering: choose meats that are grilled, poached, baked or broiled rather than fried; ask for sauces and dressings on the side; remove the bread basket from the table or take a piece and return the rest; ask for foods to be prepared without added fats, including vegetables, meats and starches like potatoes; and request smaller servings or lunch-sized portions.

After you get your meal, you can also put half of your meal in a doggie bag before beginning to eat. Trimming away visible fat and removing skin from poultry gets rid of extra, unhealthy calories. You can choose to split a meal with a friend or significant other or order from the appetizer menu only. Don't forget to drink plenty of water to help you feel full and take home your leftovers for another meal.

In addition, make mindful decisions about where you're going to eat out and how often you're going to do it. If a friend asks you to go out to dinner, you could consider asking him or her to go for a walk or just get a cup of coffee instead. You can even ask your friend over and offer to cook a healthy meal instead of eating out.

YOUR EXERCISE PLAN FOR WEEK 7

This week you get to try something new in your exercise plan: superset training. It's an advanced type of resistance work, so just plan to do it when you'll be doing one of your two or three weekly resistance training sessions. Time to get started.

WEEK 7: DIABETES BREAKTHROUGH EXERCISE PLAN

DAY	AEROBIC	RESISTANCE	STRETCHING	TYPES OF EXERCISE
1	11 minutes	30 minutes	4 minutes	Aerobic, including interval training (30-second sprints, 90 seconds of recovery)
				Resistance, including superset training (3 sets, 15 repetitions)
				Stretching

2	41 minutes		4 minutes	Aerobic, including interval training
3	11 minutes	30 minutes	4 minutes	(30-second sprints, 90 seconds of recovery)
4				Resistance, including superset training (3 sets, 15 repetitions)
5	11 minutes	30 minutes	4 minutes	Stretching
6	41 minutes		4 minutes	
7				

TOTAL TIME: 45 MINUTES

WHAT IS SUPERSET TRAINING?

This is an advanced type of strength training method in which you do two exercises, one after the other (back-to-back), with no rest in between. The exercises can be for the same muscle group or two different muscle groups. The idea is to do one exercise and, instead of resting and doing another set, doing a different exercise and alternating those exercises for your desired number of sets (usually two to three).

Benefits of Superset Training
- Total workout time is reduced while still doing the same amount of total work. If you're in a hurry in your workout, supersets can get you out of the gym faster.
- Your heart rate is elevated all the time, which improves endurance and stamina.
- Superset training recruits more muscle fibers into action, which burns more calories from glucose and fat.

EXAMPLE OF A SUPERSET TRAINING REGIMEN

Generally, you want to pair two exercises that work opposing muscle groups or areas of the body. For example, if you work your biceps (front of upper arm), you'll also need to do an exercise that works the triceps (back of upper arm); if you work your abdominal muscles, you should also do something to strengthen your lower back. Alternatively, sometimes it is beneficial to simply group exercises that work alternate parts of the body into paired activities. All of these superset exercises are paired with that principle in mind. Try doing three sets of 15 repetitions each, with no rest between alternating the following paired exercises:

- Chest press and upright rowing (see instructions for resistance training in Week 3)
- Squat and lat pull down (see resistance training in Week 3)
- High row and side-to-side steps (see circuit training in Week 4)
- Triceps press and biceps curls (see resistance training in Week 3)
- Crunches and bridging (see instructions for core stability exercises in Week 6)

STAY ACTIVE TO KEEP IT OFF

What do you think is the most effective way to lose weight and keep it off? It's the combination of changing your eating habits and being physically active. However, sticking with an exercise program can be challenging for many reasons. Since exercise is voluntary and time-consuming, it is easy to put it off or put it aside altogether when there are other important things to do. It can compete with other responsibilities and other activities that you have to do like work and family commitments.

The dropout rate from regular exercise averages 45 percent. That means that, on average, only half of the people that read this book and start exercising regularly will still be doing it a year from now. We hope that our readers beat those averages, though, and we're sure that you will. In reality, 85 percent of the Joslin Why WAIT program participants have been able to achieve the target regular exercise and to maintain it, primarily because the program progressed appropriately without causing injury or burnout and allowed them to develop a strong exercise habit along the way. In the next section, we'll talk about what you need to do to ensure you don't fall into the group that isn't exercising.

WHAT ARE THE FIVE STAGES OF PHYSICAL ACTIVITY?

The goal of this program is to help you become an active exerciser now, but your goal truly should be to be an active exerciser six months from now as well. There are five stages of change in physical activity:

1. **Couch potato/inactive:** someone who doesn't do any planned exercise (or as little as humanly possible).
2. **Inactive thinker:** "In the next six months, I'll do some exercise."
3. **Planner:** someone taking steps to be active, such as buying exercise equipment or joining a gym (but not using it much yet).
4. **Activator:** active, but not as much as probably should be, such as only three days a week for about 30 minutes.
5. **Active exerciser:** someone who exercises five days a week, for 30 minutes and has been doing so for at least six months.

Think about where you are now. Can you recognize what phase you are in? If you can stick to the plan for six months, you are an active exerciser. At this point, you're most likely an activator: perhaps you're doing three days a week and it's been less than six months since you began exercising consistently. Set up and use SMART goals to ensure that you become an active exerciser.

HOW DO YOU OVERCOME EXERCISE BARRIERS?

It's vital to have a plan to help you stay on track with your exercising if barriers arise. What issues have you had since you started this plan that made you unable to stick to the exercise plan? Perhaps you got sick or had work issues. You need to figure out a plan for how you will deal with these types of barriers to your exercise routine.

Here are some ideas of ways you can overcome some of your potential barriers to being more active. For instance, you could walk first thing in the morning to make sure that you actually do it; you could do supersets or other exercises inside if the weather is bad; or you could make exercise a social event by working out with other people. Another great thing to do if you're not feeling motivated to exercise is to tell yourself to just start with 10 minutes of activity. In most cases, by the time you've finished those 10 minutes, you'll feel better and more motivated to do the rest of your workout.

Strategies for Becoming an Active Exerciser

- Overcome any barriers you have to being active.
- Effectively manage your schedule so that you will have time to be active.
- Use your social support network to help keep you active.
- Set SMART exercise-related goals.

OUT OF TIME TO EXERCISE?

The number one reason why people don't exercise is a perceived lack of time; they think they can't fit it into their schedules. What should you do to overcome this barrier? Start by keeping track of how you exercise and think about how you might use your time more efficiently or differently to find opportunities to add in more activity easily. For example, on busy days you may want to break up your aerobic exercise session into several 10- to 15-minute bouts. If your work or other schedule makes it difficult for you to be active, having exercise equipment at home might be good for you because you can use it at any time of day. Even just having stretching bands at home is a good, affordable way to make sure that you can always get some physical activity.

Keep using your SMART goals so that you'll continue exercising when perceived time barriers arise. Remember, your goals for exercise need to be specific, measurable, adjustable, realistic and have a time frame attached. So, for example, instead of just saying, "I'll exercise more," you could say, "I will perform three sets of 15 repetitions of resistance exercises with my green bands three days a week for the next six weeks."

Sometimes the problem is not lack of time, but poor time management. Good time management involves allocating and scheduling time for exercise and setting priorities. To prevent this from being an issue, you need to look at your calendar and plan exactly when you're going to exercise, what you're going to do and for how long. Even if it's a holiday or you're busy with family and friends, you need to make some time for yourself. Make it a habit to put yourself, your health and your exercise first.

Effective Time Management
- Keep track and analyze how you use your time.
- Schedule time to exercise.
- Decide what to do with your exercise time.
- Make a commitment to your exercise time.

BREAK IT UP INTO SMALLER CHUNKS
The good news is that breaking up your workout into a few shorter sessions is as effective as completing the whole workout at once. In one study, one group of people did 40 minutes of exercise all at once while another group completed the same in four sessions throughout the day. The people who did four sessions a day for 10 minutes each actually lost more weight and did more minutes of exercise per week. A similar study in people with type 2 diabetes reported that three 10-minute walks actually controlled blood glucose levels better than a single 30-minute workout.

What's more, people who have the flexibility to do multiple sessions a day are better able to stick to their plan and, consequently, are able to do more exercise and get better results. You don't need to exercise 60 minutes in a row; you can break it up into two 30-minute sessions and burn the same amount of calories and even doing four 15-minute workouts would work. A flexible, adaptive attitude will help you fit your exercise in every day.

GET HELP FROM YOUR FAMILY AND FRIENDS
Social support is also very important to establishing new behaviors. You need to surround yourself with people who support your effort to incorporate exercise into your life, not people who will try to talk you out of it. Go walking with people you know, or maybe even make some new friends to exercise with.

Make a list of things that will help you stick to your plan and share them with family and friends. Think about all the barriers that we have discussed and how you're going to deal with them and ask family/friends for help coming up with solutions. Getting support from your family and friends in maintaining your new exercise habit is a critical part of your long-term success.

MAKE ANY GROUP WORK FOR YOU

Claudia's parting words from the Why WAIT program were "Despite many attempts to lose weight and regaining sometimes more than we lost, as a group we believed that we'd be able to end the yo-yo dieting, reach our goals, maintain our new weights and be healthier—and now we are."

Even though this book cannot take the place of doing the program in person at the Joslin Diabetes Center when it comes to the effects of group dynamics, the online social networks of people following lifestyle programs as well as people you might meet at your local gym or out in your community, will work just as well.

DIABETES BREAKTHROUGH WEEK 8

Body Core Exercises, Dining Out and
Managing Urges and Cravings

This week, we will take the time to revisit both the importance of body core training and how to manage your urges and cravings by monitoring your hunger level and other factors. Once you start to get complacent about your lifestyle changes, it's easier for things to come along and start to derail your progress. Keep vigilant and don't let that happen to you now that you're two-thirds of the way through the initial 12-week program.

This week, you'll also pick up some new skills to use when eating out at restaurants. Planning ahead and picking better foods at restaurants can help you keep your blood glucose, calorie intake and stress levels lower.

MAKE THE TIME TO REAP THE REWARDS

After many years with type 2 diabetes, Carla wasn't feeling satisfied with her body weight and her diabetes control, but everyone around her—including her husband, in-laws, friends and coworkers—seemed more concerned about her health than she was. She initially balked at joining the Joslin Why WAIT program, but finally decided to take the plunge.

"I finally made the time," she says. "I realized that if I didn't I was going to feel bad and pay for a whole lot of medications for the rest of my life. And I knew diabetes was eventually going to take its toll on my health."

BUILD A STRONG CORE

This week we're revisiting the importance of core stability training, which as an integral part of strength training will not only improve your muscle strength, but also improve your posture and reduce the risk of lower back injury. It's also a good time to revisit your target blood glucose and A1C levels and set SMART goals related to both short- and long-term goals for managing your diabetes and your weight.

WHY HAVING A STRONG CORE MATTERS

Having a strong body core is the key to being able to get around when you're older and take care of yourself. Core strength and stability training are components of physical health that often get overlooked with aging and weight gain. A recent study published in *Diabetes Care*, however, demonstrated that focusing on these components can lower the risk of falling in older people with type 2 diabetes, many of whom have some nerve damage in their feet or other health issues. After only six weeks of doing resistance and balance training, participants in that study had better balance, faster reaction times and a lesser risk of falling down. Maintaining a strong core will also help you prevent lower back pain and improve your ability to do self-care, walking and other everyday activities.

A STRONG CORE KEEPS YOU ON YOUR FEET

Most core exercises that help with stability and reduce your risk of falling as you age are done using your own body weight as resistance—no special equipment needed. By learning what exercises you can easily do on your own in the privacy of your own home, you'll be equipped to keep yourself strong and agile enough to take care of yourself throughout your lifetime. You can also lower your risk of falling down. Once you've experienced even one fall that leads to an injury, you may become less active to avoid falling again—which is totally a self-defeating strategy. The best offense in this case is to work on preserving your core strength before you ever lose it, so you can keep doing everything that you want to do during the rest of your long (and healthy) life.

YOUR EXERCISE PLAN FOR WEEK 8

Each week, your exercise should build on what you did the previous weeks—and you'll be increasing up to doing 50 minutes of exercise on five days this week. Even if we don't tell you to do every type of exercise training that you've tried so far, it never hurts to add in a variety each week. Back in Week 6, you began doing some core stability exercises as part of your training and this week you learned more about why they're so important to preventing falls and staying healthy as you age. Make sure you add some of them in this week, along with a variety of superset training (from last week), intervals, circuit training (50 seconds each and three full circuits), resistance work, aerobic training and even yoga. It never hurts to keep mixing it up for the best cross-training effect.

WEEK 8: DIABETES BREAKTHROUGH EXERCISE PLAN

DAY	AEROBIC	RESISTANCE	STRETCHING	TYPES OF EXERCISE
1	11 minutes	35 minutes	4 minutes	Aerobic, including interval training
2	46 minutes		4 minutes	(40-second sprints, 1 minute and 20 seconds of recovery)
3	11 minutes	35 minutes	4 minutes	Resistance, including circuit
4				training (50 seconds at each station, 3 circuits)
5	11 minutes	35 minutes	4 minutes	Stretching
6	46 minutes		4 minutes	
7				

TOTAL TIME: 50 MINUTES

DINING OUT WITH DIABETES

The average American eats away from home about four times per week. Maintaining good blood glucose control and eating heart-healthy is a challenge in a restaurant, but it can be done. Although it would be unreasonable to expect you never to eat out, try your best to limit the number of meals you eat outside your house.

When you do go out, remember that you're not a victim in a restaurant; you're a paying customer. There are noticeable changes happening in terms of the amount and types of foods that restaurants serve and these adaptations are probably the result of concerned consumers making suggestions. In the meantime, it's up to you to practice portion control, choose healthier foods and time your meal so that it works properly with your medications.

Keep in mind some of the pitfalls and you can learn some of the questions to ask when eating out. The following are some of the challenges we face when dining out:

- You are not doing the cooking and can't see what or how much is being added to your meal. The fat, sodium or carbohydrate content is often unknown (and usually one or more are higher than you would normally choose to eat).
- Fat is flavor and is very often added to give foods a rich flavor or textures that are flaky, crispy or creamy.
- Salt is the number one spice that most chefs use to bring out flavor in food and very often you may not even notice that a food tastes salty.
- Portions are too big and oversized portions have become the standard in restaurants today. Even if you try to eat less, you may still be eating more than you would at home.
- Meat is the entrée. Meat, specifically red meat, can be high in calories because it usually takes up more than half of the dinner plate. To stay healthy, our bodies need less than half the protein that restaurants serve and a whole lot less fat.
- You may think of a meal away from home as a special occasion. Years ago you may have only eaten out on birthdays or special

occasions. If you eat out often, you need to be more mindful of what you are ordering.

Actions You Can Take When Eating Out
- Trim away visible fat from meat.
- Remove skin from poultry.
- Split your meal with your dining companion.
- Order an appetizer or two rather than a full entrée.
- Drink plenty of water with your meal.
- Take home leftovers.

PLANNING AHEAD HELPS WITH YOUR MEDICATIONS

When going out to eat, plan what you will eat and when you will take your medication. If you eat out spontaneously, there's a chance that you won't make the best dietary decisions. However, if you plan ahead, you're much more likely to make better decisions. Find out where you're going to eat and with whom. If you know where you're going, look at the menu online before you go; a lot of restaurants have nutritional information available on their websites. If a restaurant doesn't, email them and say that you're going to their restaurant and want to know their nutritional information.

Consider the timing of your medications. Think about when you're going to be taking your insulin, Byetta, Victoza, Symlin or pills that have a specific effect related to a meal. Plan ahead so that you don't either have to forego taking it or take it too soon and suffer from low blood glucose. If you take fast-acting insulin like Novolog, Humalog or Apidra, you should wait at least until you actually see your meal before you take your insulin. As mentioned before, to enhance how much weight you lose, you may need to take your insulin dose immediately after a meal based on what you actually ate instead of before. You have a window of 20 minutes from your first bite, whether you start with an appetizer, soup or salad, to inject your rapid-acting insulin. If you delay the injection more than that, you may get hypoglycemia later than two hours after eating. You should inject Symlin about 10 to 15 minutes before the meal, but don't take it much before then or else it may make you feel nauseated. The further away from the meal you take the Byetta—up until an hour before—the better it will work for suppressing your appetite, but you must take it within an hour before eating for it to be effective.

A GUIDE TO HEALTHY CHOICES WHEN DINING OUT

The following provides a guide to eating out in various restaurants and a list of tips to help you ask the right questions and make healthy choices when eating out.

TYPE OF RESTAURANT	FOODS TO CHOOSE	FOODS TO AVOID	ORDERING TIPS
European	Clear broth or consommé with noodles or vegetables; Cornish game hens prepared without fat, skin removed; poached, steamed or boiled entrées	Goose or duck, cream soups, croissants, pastry/pastry shells, sauces	Choose restaurants that serve nouvelle French or California cuisine Ask for sauces on the side Ask for foods to be sautéed in broth rather than butter
Middle Eastern	Pita bread, stuffed grape leaves, tandoori chicken, curries made without coconut milk, rice, yogurt, chutneys, tabouli	Most lamb dishes, breads made with or cooked in butter, fried falafel	Ask for vegetarian versions of dishes Ask if chicken or fish can be substituted for lamb or beef
Mexican	Steamed corn tortillas with salsa, chicken tostado, burrito without cheese, fish dishes, chicken fajitas	Tortilla chips; beef and cheese burritos; fried and refried foods, such as refried beans	Ask for foods to be prepared without sour cream or cheese Use guacamole sparingly

Italian	Pasta with marinara or clam sauce, pizza with vegetable toppings, veal with tomato sauce, minestrone soup	Pasta with cream sauces, pizza with meat toppings, extra cheese	Choose dishes prepared with red sauce Ask for foods to be sautéed in wine and lemon juice instead of butter
Asian	Steamed vegetarian dumplings, steamed rice, noodle dishes that aren't fried, chicken or fish dishes that are steamed, stir-fried or broiled vegetarian dishes, hot and sour soups, fortune cookies	Egg rolls and other fried appetizers, breaded or deep-fried dishes, duck, fried rice, spare ribs	Choose steamed dishes rather than fried Ask if dishes can be prepared with less oil
American	Plain baked potato or sweet potato with margarine, steamed vegetables, salads, grilled or broiled poultry, fish or lean meat (loin or round choices)	Cheeseburgers, fish burgers, fried chicken, French fries, milkshakes, cream sauces and gravies	Look for lower-fat, healthier options when eating at fast-food restaurants

Adapted from Joslin Diabetes Center education materials.
Copyright © 2012 by Joslin Diabetes Center (www.joslin.org). All rights reserved.

DRINK ALCOHOL IN MODERATION ONLY

Alcohol is another issue that comes along with eating out and socializing in general and it can be a source of lapses or slips. Your body sees alcohol as a toxin, so your liver tries to metabolize it to get rid of it, making it so busy that it doesn't release as much stored glucose. If you haven't eaten and choose to drink alcohol, your blood glucose can get too low. When that happens, you'll likely eat more than you planned to.

In addition, be sure your blood glucose is in good control before you drink. Liquor doesn't have any carbohydrates and wine has only a minimal amount (depending on its residual sugar content), so they don't affect blood glucose that much except if you haven't eaten. Beer, on the other hand, does have carbohydrates. All alcohol is full of empty calories and also stimulates appetite. More important, it can also lower inhibitions with regard to keeping your diabetes in check. For example, drinking may cause you to let your guard down and eat something that you otherwise wouldn't.

Remember that a drink is a 5-ounce glass of wine, 12 ounces of beer or 1.5 ounces of liquor, all of which have about 100 calories coming from the alcohol alone, making drinks packed full of empty calories. A typical bottle of wine (750 ml) contains about five glasses containing five ounces each. If you use mixers or drink wine coolers, you have to take the added carbohydrate and calories into account, as well.

Moderation is the key, both for your health in general and specifically for maintaining blood glucose control. Check with your doctor first, but drinking a limited amount of alcohol is generally okay when you have diabetes. Just make sure you always have alcohol on a full stomach. You really should never have more than one (for women) to two (for men) drinks per day and limiting yourself to two to three days per week is recommended. Alcohol can also affect your triglycerides (blood fats), so limit drinking if those are already high.

Healthy Tips for Dining Out
PLAN AHEAD

- Choose restaurants that offer healthy menu choices.
- Collect menus from your favorite restaurants to help you plan your selections ahead of time.
- Look online for restaurant nutrition information either using the restaurant's own website or sites like www.dietfacts.com or www.calorieking.com.
- Call the restaurants ahead of time to ask about portions and preparation.

CONTROL PORTIONS

- Ask the server not to bring the bread basket, or take one piece and ask for the bread basket to be removed.
- Know your meal plan or carry a copy on a small card with you.
- Ask the server to pack up part of your meal before it's served.
- Share an entrée with your spouse or friend.
- Order from the appetizer menu (soup or salad) in place of an entrée.
- Stay away from buffets or all-you-can-eat specials if portion control is a problem for you.

MAKE REQUESTS

- If you're unsure about ingredients or how foods are prepared, ask.
- Ask if your meal can be grilled or poached instead of fried, or prepared without added fat.
- Ask that sauces, dressings and gravies be served on the side; use sparingly.
- Find out if low-calorie salad dressings, skim milk or fresh fruit options are available.

TIMING

- Consider the timing of your insulin or diabetes medication.
- If your meal will be later, eat a small snack at your usual mealtime to avoid a low blood glucose.
- If you take pills or fast-acting insulin, you can take them after you get to the restaurant in case your meal is served late.
- Talk to your health care provider about varying the dose and timing of your insulin if restaurant meal times are different from your usual mealtimes.
- Check your blood glucose more often whenever you eat meals at different times.

ALCOHOL

- Alcohol can put you at risk for low blood glucose if taken on an empty stomach; try to wait and have an alcoholic beverage with your meal.
- Alcohol does stimulate appetite and often people will eat more than planned.

continued

IF YOU OVEREAT

- Check your blood glucose more often.
- Take a walk or do some exercise.
- Get back on track at the next meal.
- Don't skip your next meal to compensate.
- Don't give up; think about what you might do differently next time.

MANAGING URGES AND CRAVINGS

Often motivators other than hunger can drive our eating, including smell, sight, habit and cravings. Let's talk first about the difference between hunger and cravings. In general, physical hunger is gradual or slow in onset and feels like a gnawing in the stomach. Sometimes, hunger can cause people to feel light-headed or spacey or that food of any kind will relieve it. Cravings, on the other hand, may feel sudden in onset, more on a conscious level. You may feel it in your mouth or in your thoughts and you will usually crave specific foods, such as sweet or salty ones.

In order to tell the difference between hunger and a craving, you have to know what being hungry feels like to you. Hunger isn't connected to an on-off switch; there are different levels of hunger. That may seem obvious to you if you are more in touch with your feelings of hunger, but not if you bounce from starving to stuffed all day.

A hunger scale can be a useful tool to help you avoid overeating. Your dietary logbook has a column labeled Hunger Level that has been asking you to rate your hunger on a scale of 1 to 5, where 1 is "starved" and 5 is "stuffed." But what's in between and where should you stop?

At the end of a meal or snack, your goal should be to land somewhere around a 3 (comfortable) or a 4 (full). You don't want to let yourself get overly hungry (below a 2, or hungry) because that's where you are likely to start feeling the more uncomfortable feelings of hunger that can lead you to overeat. You would definitely not want to eat to above a 4, either, the point where you feel full. So practice using this scale to get more in touch with how hungry or full you feel and aim to stop eating at a 3 or 4.

Be sure to keep recording your hunger or fullness levels in your logbook. By doing so, you'll learn how to stop when you're no more than 80 percent full to give your food time to settle. Remember, it takes a full 15 to 20 minutes for your stomach to send the signal to your brain that it is full. If you eat until you're full, you will likely feel more than full by the time your brain gets that signal.

Use the Hunger Scale

1. Rate your hunger on a scale of 1–5 before you eat.

2. Halfway through your meal, stop eating and rate your hunger again.

3. Stop eating if you rate 3 or above.

4. Rate your hunger level 20 minutes after you eat. Are you comfortable? Full? Stuffed?

5. Use alternate activities (like those introduced in Week 4) if you are tempted to keep eating when you're above 4.

RATE YOUR HUNGER

1	2	3	4	5
Starved	Hungry	Comfortable	Full	Stuffed

If hunger and fullness were the only regulators of eating, people would not struggle with weight. But we don't always eat when we are hungry and stop when we're full. There are many emotional and social aspects to our eating patterns, as well. An important question to ask yourself before you eat is, "What am I really hungry for?" If you are actually tired, lonely, sad or some other emotion, then food is not really the solution to that particular problem and you need to find a different coping strategy (for which you may need to revisit the delay and distraction strategies that were introduced during Week 4). For example, if you are tired, get some rest instead of eating. Likewise, if you are lonely, find a way to connect with other people instead of turning to food to make you feel better.

On the other hand, if you have checked in with yourself and established that you are hungry or you want to respond to a craving, then you should go ahead and eat. It's not bad to eat something simply because you crave it, but you want to be sure that you don't overeat it. Use the same hunger scale when you're eating a craved food, too, to avoid doing just that.

Tips for Managing Cravings
- Aim to outlast the urge—delay, delay, delay.
- Set a kitchen timer or your watch for a set amount of time.
- Use delay, distraction and alternative coping strategies (see Week 4 for tips).
- Ask yourself, "What am I really hungry for?" and then try to solve the underlying problem:
  - Am I really lonely?
  - Am I bored and need a purpose?
  - Am I upset or stressed?
  - Am I tired and need to relax?
  - Is it a habit?

TAKE CHARGE OF YOUR DIABETES AND YOUR LIFE

Although she put off starting it for a considerable amount of time, Carla recalls, "After spending 12 weeks with the Why WAIT program, I wonder why I waited so long to do this. I lost 25 pounds and have a renewed sense of life. I'm also more proactive about my health." She has continued practicing her new lifestyle with success and she tells anyone who will listen that she's now in charge of her diabetes instead of the reverse. Are you?

DIABETES BREAKTHROUGH WEEK 9

Mental Stress, Deep Breathing and Relaxation Exercises

We'll shift your focus a bit this week to managing your mental stress, which is a key part of both weight loss and effective blood glucose control. You'll learn some breathing and relaxation techniques that will help you deal with daily stressors, improving your blood glucose control and how much weight you lose. Even if you haven't joined the yoga craze, it's possible to use progressive muscle and other relaxation techniques to effectively relieve stress.

LOSE THE DIABETES STRESS

Getting complications from diabetes was Susan's biggest worry in life—and she spent a lot of time getting new wrinkles and gray hairs over it. Although she'd done everything possible to keep her blood glucose levels in check, she had just about given up hope that she'd ever really be the master over them. However, after she finished the Joslin Why WAIT program, things had dramatically changed for her. We'll tell you more later about how she finally was able to stop worrying so much.

STRESS, BE GONE

Why does stress matter so much? Not only can it cause you to give in to your urges (i.e., emotional eating), but stress alone can sabotage your attempts to lose weight and lower your insulin needs. You can lower your stress by managing guilt stemming from making unhealthy choices when you eat out. What's more, there's a physical component that also needs to be managed.

Mental stress actually elevates levels of a natural hormone called cortisol and higher secretion of that hormone can make you get more belly fat. A recent study in the *Journal of Obesity* examined what happens when overweight and obese women practice mindful eating and relaxation skills and the results were encouraging. Four months of practice with mindfulness lowered their stress levels, cortisol and bad abdominal fat—and you'll learn more about how to eat mindfully next week.

Even in preteens, higher levels of cortisol in the morning have been linked to bigger waistlines, according to an article in *Journal of Pediatric Endocrinology and Metabolism*. Luckily for you, this program is designed to help you naturally lower your stress levels and the hormone that prevents you from losing weight and increases your fasting blood glucose.

MANAGE YOUR STRESS TO BETTER MANAGE YOUR LIFE

Stress is an inevitable part of all of our lives, but it does not have to rule your life or sabotage your weight loss attempts or your blood glucose control. This week, we're going to focus on stress and its impact on weight loss and maintenance. Unfortunately, many people often turn to food for comfort during times of stress. Thus, adopting coping strategies for stress management that are not food-related is key to successful weight loss.

Let's start with mental stress. What are some of the things that make you feel stressed? How do you know when you're stressed? For most people, certain specific situations cause stress. You might also start to get some bodily cues that tell you you're stressed: your heart starts pounding or you get a headache or muscle tension in your neck, shoulders and back. This is helpful information because in order for you to manage stress you first need to identify those situations that cause you stress and how you react.

Recognize Your Unique Stress Signals

- Do you get sweaty? Short of breath? A headache? An upset stomach?
- Are you cranky? Irritable?
- Do you stay in bed? Have trouble sleeping?
- Do you overeat?
- Do you lose your appetite?

What do you currently do to manage your stress? What other means (other than eating) can you use to manage stressful feelings and situations? How will you reward yourself when you feel you deserve a treat or need comfort?

You can try a whole body approach through yoga, meditation or progressive muscle relaxation exercises. Exercise is also an important tool to manage stress. Gentle, slow movement like yoga and stretching can be really helpful for some people, while others prefer to de-stress with more vigorous activity such as walking or swimming or other types of aerobic exercise. One way that exercise helps with stress is by making you take deeper breaths, which brings more oxygen to your muscles and can help them relax. This kind of deep breathing is also what happens naturally as our bodies shift from being awake to sleeping.

Take Action to Decrease Your Stress

- Breathe deeply and slowly. How we breathe can make us feel better or worse. When you notice you are breathing fast, pay attention to your breaths:
  - Let your lower abdomen extend out as you breathe in through your nose to a count of five.
  - Hold the breath for a count of five.
  - Blow out through your mouth for a count of five.
  - If a count of five feels too long, then do it for as long as you can or pick a count that feels comfortable to you.

continued

- Avoid negative people. Try to surround yourself with people who make you feel good about yourself. Talk to calm people when you feel stressed.

- Look for the humor in life. A good laugh physically relaxes tense muscles.

- Learn to say "no." Lots of people make demands on us. Do you really want to do it and do you have the time? Let yourself cancel plans if you should have declined when you said "yes."

RELIEVE STRESS WITH RELAXATION

Practicing yoga or other relaxation techniques like meditation may have more health benefits than you realize. For starters, doing any activity that helps reduce your stress levels can automatically lower levels of the stress hormone cortisol associated not only with weight gain, but also with high morning blood glucose. By controlling cortisol and stress levels naturally with relaxation techniques of any type, you will drop excess weight faster and impress your doctor with your excellent blood glucose. Yoga can help prevent low-back pain as well and being more flexible decreases your risk of getting injured during physical activities.

RESTING DEEP-BREATHING EXERCISE

Try taking a few deep breaths right now. Stay seated in a chair, get comfortable and just close your eyes. Tune into your breathing: don't change it, just notice each breath in and each breath out. Focus on just your breathing for 20 to 30 seconds. Then slowly take a deep breath in . . . hold it . . . and exhale slowly . . . again . . . and one last time.

A simple deep breathing exercise like that can be a great way to de-stress anytime, at work or whenever you notice that you're feeling stressed.

Relax Using Other Senses (Besides Taste)

TOUCH

- Try stretching and massage.
- Treat yourself to a manicure.
- Cozy up on the couch with a snuggly blanket.

SMELL

- Concentrate on slowing down your breathing and relaxing.
- Burn a nicely scented candle.
- Light a fire in the fireplace.
- Use a lotion with a fragrance you like.

HEARING

- Listen to relaxing music.
- Go to a concert.
- Turn off the TV, radio and phone and enjoy the quiet.

SEEING

- Get out of the house and exercise.
- Surround yourself with beauty.
- Buy yourself something nice and new.

YOUR EXERCISE PLAN FOR WEEK 9

In addition to adding in a sixth day of exercise this week, you'll also be adding in some mixed interval and superset training at least one day this week. It's not too tricky—just find ways to combine some of your supersets (discussed in Week 7) with some intervals, either during aerobic sets or using circuits. In addition, to help you manage your stress, you'll be trying out some progressive muscle relaxation and other de-stressing exercises.

WEEK 9: DIABETES BREAKTHROUGH EXERCISE PLAN

DAY	AEROBIC	RESISTANCE	STRETCHING	TYPES OF EXERCISE
1	10 minutes	40 minutes	5 minutes	Aerobic, including interval training
2	50 minutes		5 minutes	Resistance, including superset training
3	10 minutes	40 minutes	5 minutes	(2 sets, 15 repetitions) Stretching
4				
5	50 minutes		5 minutes	
6	10 minutes	40 minutes	5 minutes	
7	50 minutes		5 minutes	

TOTAL TIME: 55 MINUTES

ADDITIONAL EXERCISES FOR MIXED INTERVAL AND SUPERSET TRAINING

1. **QUADRICEPS—Lunge Step (Backward)**

   Standing in a stride stance, anchor the resistance band under your forward foot. Keep your palms forward at shoulder height. Step back with your other leg, allowing it to flex. Make sure that your knees are not moving forward above your toes. Repeat with your other leg. If you find this exercise challenging and feel pain in your knees, hips or lower back, you should avoid doing it.

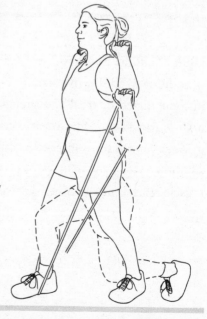

2. SHOULDERS—Alternate Front Arm Raise

Anchor resistance band under your feet. Palms down, raise one arm to shoulder height while breathing out. Breathe in while returning back to the starting position and alternate with your other arm. If limited in range of motion, raise your arm only halfway or as far as possible. If you find this exercise challenging and feel pain in your neck or shoulders, you should avoid doing it.

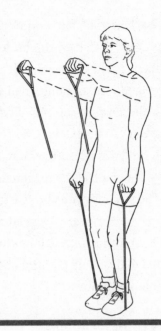

PROGRESSIVE MUSCLE RELAXATION EXERCISE

Let's try a technique called progressive muscle relaxation that you can do whenever you have time. After you turn down the lights (but not off), get comfortable in your seat by uncrossing your legs, placing your feet flat on the floor and putting your hands in your lap. The rest of this exercise should take about eight minutes to complete (from toe to head).

Close your eyes if that's comfortable and start by focusing on your breathing, slowing down your breathing, inhaling and exhaling. Bring your attention to your feet and notice any tension in them. Tense your feet as much as you can and curl your toes and your arches. Focus on tensing them as much as you can, but make sure you're not holding your breath. Release the tension, return to doing slow, deep breathing and notice how your feet feel. Do the same thing with your legs, by tightening the muscles of your calves and thighs as much as you can—really tightly—and then release. Make sure you breathe throughout the contraction and return to doing deep breathing.

The rest of this exercise progresses next to your trunk, back, neck, shoulders, arms, hands and finally your face, tensing muscles and then relaxing them, always returning to some deep breathing in between tensing up a different part of your body.

Start back at your feet and notice and release any tension there. Move up to your ankles, calves, thighs, lower back, abdomen, mid- and upper back, shoulders, neck, jaw, forehead, checks and all the muscles in your face. Take a deep breath in and out when you're focusing on each individual area and release the tension there. Finally, take a few more deep breaths and when you're ready, you can open your eyes.

How did this relaxation exercise make you feel? Did your breathing change? Where did you feel the most tension? Just becoming conscious of where you hold the stress in your body can help you to release it. Do this exercise on your own whenever you need to relax. In addition, practice deep breathing or the other relaxations throughout the day whenever you're feeling stressed. Take some additional time to practice the full progressive muscle relaxation technique.

RELAXATION TECHNIQUES

Relaxations are a great tool to use to manage stress during times when you may have just a few minutes to relax. Try each of the methods below and use the one that works best for you whenever you need a break from stress. Some people like to alternate, using a slightly different technique each time they practice.

1. Before you start, think of a "focus word" that makes you feel calm and relaxed. Some people like to use a word that describes a feeling (serene), the word *breathe* or simply a sound *(om)*. Once you've selected your word, take a deep breath and hold it for a few seconds. Then repeat your focus word as you let your breath out very slowly.

2. Put one hand just under your navel (belly button). Focus on breathing deeply into your abdomen so that your hand rises when you breathe in and falls when you exhale. Now, as you inhale, say the number 10 to yourself. Exhale. With the next inhalation, say the number nine and then breathe out. Do not speed up your breathing—continue with regular deep breaths. Continue to slowly count inhalations until you reach zero.

3. Put your hand on your abdomen just under your navel. As you breathe in count slowly up: one, two, three, four. As you exhale, count very slowly back down: four, three, two, one.

4. Breathe in through your nose and then breathe out through your mouth. Notice how cool the air feels as you inhale in contrast to how warm it feels when you exhale. Continue breathing slowly, noticing your breath each time you inhale and exhale.

Adapted from *Self-Nurture* by Alice Domar, Ph.D. (Penguin Books, 2001).

LOSE THE STRESS TO BE HEALTHY

Remember Susan's gray hairs and wrinkle lines coming from worrying about getting diabetes-related complications? Sometimes just gaining knowledge can be a powerful tool in reducing your need to worry.

Susan says, "For me, the Why WAIT program brought home how closely eating and exercise are related, not just when it comes to lowering blood glucose, but for being healthy in general. Through the tools I gained, I know it's now within my power to control my diabetes and stay healthy." That peace of mind alone helps keep her stress down and blood glucose levels in check. Is it working for you yet?

DIABETES BREAKTHROUGH WEEK 10

Mindful Eating, Sleep and Balance and Agility Exercises

As far as your diet is concerned this week, you'll be focusing on learning to eat mindfully, how that is key to keeping your diet on track and how coping with stress cuts down on emotional eating. You'll also learn why sleep matters to weight loss. The new exercise you'll be doing this week also incorporates some balance and agility training that will enhance both your balance and your fitness gains. The knowledge you are acquiring through this program is certain to make your physical and mental rewards ongoing.

PROVE IT, PLEASE
A scientist by training, 55-year-old Regina wanted to be convinced that the Joslin Why WAIT program was scientifically proven before she started it. Testimonials just didn't cut it for her. She had to see it to believe it. So, she waded through all the research articles that Dr. Hamdy's group had published about past participants before joining. The evidence she saw was enough to persuade her to give the program a try. We'll tell you later, though, why she's now giving a testimonial—something that she didn't believe in before.

LEARN HOW TO EAT MINDFULLY, NOT EMOTIONALLY

If you want to effectively modify your diet for a lifetime, you need to learn how to eat mindfully, as has been demonstrated by many studies including a study in *Complementary Therapies in Medicine*. In that study, when ten individuals were trained in mindfulness, meditation and mindful eating, they increased their awareness of bodily sensations, emotions and triggers that normally made them overeat. As a result, they all found it easier to have more control around food, their weight went down and they experienced less depression, binge eating and stress. What's not to like about that?

Many prior studies on mindful eating have also shown that being aware of what you're eating allows you to make better choices about what and how much you consume. Instead of telling you to avoid all situations in which eating may be a problem for you, we take the approach that you need to learn how to make informed choices about intake of fat, carbohydrates, sodium and other nutrients that can impact your body weight, blood glucose and health. Being mindful means you'll consciously eat less and pick foods that are better for you.

LEARN HOW TO PRACTICE MINDFUL EATING

This week, you get to practice eating with awareness, otherwise known as *mindful eating*. Being mindful in this case means eating on a conscious level: being actively aware of what, why and how you're eating. Your emphasis is on enjoying the food as a fully sensual experience and not clouding the experience by shame, guilt or other negative emotions.

This concept applies to all eating, but it can be an especially helpful approach when you're eating a craved food. The conscious choice to eat a food that you're craving often involves feeling guilty and playing a lot of mental games like rationalizing what you're doing or looking at it in black-and-white terms like we have already discussed (such as "If I am going to blow it, I may as well have a lot of it since I won't ever be eating this again").

To change this kind of attitude toward food and eating, start thinking about the big picture. Food should be a pleasure, not a source of stress. If you're going to have something that is not on the meal plan, then focus first on establishing a reasonable portion and next on really enjoying the experience of eating it. In addition, make sure that you only facilitate eating it that one time. For instance, if you choose to have ice cream, buy only a small kiddie cone or have a reasonable serving at an ice cream shop rather than having extra ice cream left over in your freezer to tempt you at a later time.

Try this exercise at home. Get a bag of raisins or Hershey's Kisses® or M&M'S®—and take just one of them out of the bag and eat it, focusing on really experiencing it. Notice its texture, smell and taste as you chew it slowly. What do you notice about the food when you do this?

Snacking is one area that many people have a problem with when it comes to eating mindfully. For example, previous Why WAIT participants have shared that they've polished off a large bag of chips or a whole carton of ice cream without even realizing it while watching television. You really need to practice being more mindful when snacking.

One suggestion on how to do this includes ritualizing snacking; for example, having tea and a snack every day at three in the afternoon and not doing anything else while you are doing it except for really focusing on the experience. Making food into an enjoyable ritual like this helps you to eat more slowly and more consciously. You can also make your snacking more conscious by turning off the TV and sitting at the kitchen table to eat a snack. In short, get rid of all the distractions you can and just focus on savoring each bite of your food.

Tips for Practicing Mindful Eating

- Pick a mealtime and an eating place where you won't be disturbed.
- Serve food in attractive plates and bowls.
- Before eating, take one to two minutes to breathe deeply and relax.
- Ask yourself why you are eating.
- Make sure you really want the food you are eating.
- Take less food than you think you need.
- Look at the food and notice colors and textures.
- Smell the food and inhale the aroma.
- Taste the food, savoring it.
- Chew thoroughly and eat slowly.
- Put your fork down between bites of food and breathe as you eat.

continued

- Resolve to relax after you're done eating.
- Wait 20 minutes before making any decisions about going back for seconds.

WHAT TO DO IF YOU OVEREAT

It's normal to slip up and eat too much sometimes. The important thing is to get back on track right away if you do have a slip. Now that you are starting to understand more about the distribution of calories in your meal plan, you understand what the numbers mean. So if you look at a cookie and see it's 400 calories, you will realize that you could spend your whole lunch's worth of calories on one cookie. However, these are decisions you have to learn to manage for yourself. If you want the cookie that badly, have it. There's room for flexibility.

Being successful at weight loss over the long-term means moving away from black-and-white thinking. If you do choose to have the cookie, think about what you could do to help minimize its impact. Could you increase your exercise that day? Choose a smaller cookie with fewer calories the next time? Don't beat yourself up over it. Think about what your support system would say to you if you had a slip. If you feel bad, call someone, talk it through and write it in your logbook.

WHY SLEEP MATTERS TO WEIGHT LOSS

Mindful eating may also be related to how much and how well you sleep. Researchers have looked at levels of two hormones called leptin and ghrelin with regard to how much sleep people get. Leptin is a hormone that tells your brain that you're full and don't need any food. Ghrelin tells it that you're in starvation mode or that you're hungry. People who sleep only four hours have a high level of ghrelin and eat more. Those who sleep eight hours have higher levels of leptin and aren't as hungry. What these findings mean to you is that if you have sleep issues, try to get them worked out because they could impede your weight loss.

Another study followed two groups of people, one where the participants slept four hours each night and one where they slept eight hours a night, to see the effects on their blood glucose control. The people who sleep only four hours gain weight and experience worse blood glucose control. Similarly, if you don't sleep enough, your body will be in a state of stress and release stress hormones like cortisol that will trigger your liver to produce more glucose, thereby raising your blood glucose levels. That's just one more compelling reason to focus on getting enough sleep every day.

YOUR EXERCISE PLAN FOR WEEK 10

Your exercise goal for this week is to continue bumping up your training time by another five minutes on the six days you are active this week. Try some yoga again this week and practice core exercises, which will also improve your balance and are guaranteed to help you stay on your feet (especially as you continue to get older).

WEEK 10: DIABETES BREAKTHROUGH EXERCISE PLAN

DAY	AEROBIC	RESISTANCE	STRETCHING	TYPES OF EXERCISE
1	15 minutes	40 minutes	5 minutes	Aerobic, including interval training
2	55 minutes		5 minutes	Resistance, including core stability and yoga
3	15 minutes	40 minutes	5 minutes	Stretching
4				
5	55 minutes		5 minutes	
6	15 minutes	40 minutes	5 minutes	
7	55 minutes		5 minutes	
TOTAL TIME: 60 MINUTES				

BALANCE AND AGILITY TRAINING

As soon as you pass the age of 30, other types of physical activity become more important as well, particularly exercises that help you maintain your balance and improve your posture. These can become even more important if you have developed any loss of sensation in your feet that can affect how well you can feel the ground when you walk.

When was the last time you practiced balancing on one leg for a minute or two? Poor balance is readily apparent if you try to balance by standing on one leg and shut your eyes (do this while holding on to something to be safe). You may be surprised how much worse your balance is with your eyes closed. The bad news is that your balancing ability begins to deteriorate starting around the age of 40 and poor balance is associated with an increase in falls and injuries like wrist and hip fractures. The good news is that you can regain a lot of your ability to balance simply by practicing.

To balance effectively, you need adequate strength in your ankle and hip muscles, good feedback from the nerves in your feet (to help your brain with its position sense) and a functioning brain (specifically the region called the cerebellum). Most people start to rely more heavily on their vision to compensate for negative changes in their ability to balance over time. Regardless of your age, if you can't stand steadily on one leg for at least 15 seconds—with or without your eyes closed—then you definitely need to start practicing as soon as possible to improve your balance.

The ancient Chinese exercise form known as Tai Chi is excellent for improving balance, which is not surprising given that it's the foundation of all martial arts forms. Getting involved in Tai Chi or any form of martial arts training will allow you to practice your balance while gaining lower body strength. Lower-body resistance training also doubles as balance exercise. When you do your regular strength exercises, your balance should improve at the same time. Yoga, while a lower intensity activity, can help your balance improve as well since it works on the endurance of muscles involved in your body core.

Everyday, Anytime Balance Exercises

The following exercises will improve your balance. You can do them almost anytime and as often as you like, as long as you have something sturdy nearby to hold on to as needed.

- **Stand on one leg.** To do this, hold on to a table with both hands while standing on one leg, with your eyes open. Once you're stable, slowly release one hand or both and try to stay balanced for as long as possible. Repeat with the other leg. For best results, do this exercise two to three times a day using alternating feet.

- **Challenge yourself on one leg.** The one-legged exercise can improve your balance further if you use more advanced balance techniques as you progress: (1) holding on with only one fingertip to start; (2) not holding on at all; and (3) if very steady on your feet, closing your eyes (still without holding on). Be sure to have someone stand close by in case you ever feel unsteady, especially with your eyes closed.

- **Grab a towel with your toes.** Place a towel on the floor and practice grabbing it with the toes of both of your feet, alternately, while sitting and then while standing.

- **Stand on a cushion.** Use cushions or pillows of varying firmness. Put them on the floor and stand on them with your legs alternately together and farther apart.

- **Stand with a changed position.** Try standing on two legs under different conditions: with your eyes open or closed, head tilted to one side or straight, talking or silent and hands at your sides or held out from your body.

- **Walk heel-to-toe.** Position your heel just in front of the toes of the opposite foot each time you take a step. Your heel and toes should touch or come close. You may want to begin doing this exercise following along handrails or with a wall next to you, just in case you start to feel unsteady.

- **Walk backward.** Try walking backward along a wall or a kitchen counter without looking back, using the wall or counter to steady yourself (as infrequently as possible).

A BELIEVER EVEN WITHOUT THE SCIENCE

After finishing the 12 weeks of the program, Regina was a true believer even without the research to back up the results. She recalls when the mental switch happened for her, "As the members of my Why WAIT group lost weight, we not only saw the numbers on the scale go down, but our blood glucose, blood pressure and lipid panels also followed suit."

But for her, what mattered most was that this program ended up being a life-altering experience. She says, "I never did before, but now I'm taking full responsibility for my own health and am self-motivated to keep it up. It doesn't get better than that." We have to agree with her and we hope you do, as well.

DIABETES BREAKTHROUGH WEEK 11

Secrets of Successful Losers, the Importance of Exercise and Lapse and Relapse

---

You're nearing the end of the formal 12-week Diabetes Breakthrough program, but there's still a lot left for you to learn that will help you reverse weight gain and diabetes for the rest of your life. You'll come to understand the difference between a lapse and a relapse when it comes to successful weight loss and preventing weight regain. You'll also benefit from finding out how to prevent yourself from gaining weight back by finding out how other successful "losers" have done it.

FIRST OVERWEIGHT, THEN DIABETES

After a decades-long struggle with her body weight and many unsuccessful attempts keeping the weight off after being on diet after diet, 70-year-old Velda was even more discouraged when her doctor diagnosed her with type 2 diabetes several years ago.

"I've never been thin, but somehow I just never thought I'd get diabetes," she says. Now she wonders what's in store for her health next. Luckily, she found the Joslin Why WAIT program and started down the right path at the age of 70—which shows that it's never too late to change your direction toward permanent weight loss and better health. Later, you'll hear more about how her struggles with her weight and her health are progressing now.

THE SCIENCE BEHIND SUCCESSFUL "LOSERS"

Have you heard of the National Weight Control Registry (NWCR, online at www.nwcr.ws)? Many research studies have supported exercise as a way to maintain weight loss, but the NWCR, with thousands of participants, has had dramatic results. It was established in 1994 to determine what behaviors are common in people who have lost at least 30 pounds and kept it off for at least a year (confirmed by their medical records).

It now includes over 10,000 individuals with an average weight loss of 66 pounds maintained for over five years. Women make up 80 percent of individuals in the registry and 20 percent are men. The average woman is 45 years of age and currently weighs 145 pounds, while the average man is 49 and weighs 190 pounds.

Within these averages lies a lot of diversity, though. Weight losses have ranged from 30 to 300 pounds and the duration of successful weight maintenance ranges from one year to 66 years. Some have lost the weight rapidly, while others have lost weight very slowly (e.g., over 14 years). Just over half (55 percent) used some type of weight loss program to help them and the others lost weight on their own.

EXERCISE, EXERCISE, EXERCISE

While the registry members lost the weight many different ways, almost all of them keep it off using similar techniques—one of which is exercise, an average of 60 minutes daily. It is particularly interesting to note what the people in the registry do for exercise. Walking is the preferred activity in combination with some other kind of exercise (like swimming, strength training, group classes) for 49 percent of those successful "losers," 28 percent choose to only walk, 14 percent do other exercise (strength exercises, group classes) and only 9 percent choose not to exercise. In total, 91 percent of them exercise regularly and only 9 percent don't—that should tell you something.

Exercise Data from the National Weight Control Registry

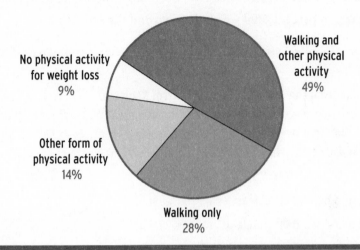

No physical activity
for weight loss
9%

Walking and
other physical
activity
49%

Other form of
physical activity
14%

Walking only
28%

In the latest NWCR research published recently in *Obesity,* people in the NWCR engage in more sustained exercise (about 41 minutes at a time) that is moderate or vigorous in nature—like brisk walking or jogging—than people who are overweight that haven't lost or kept weight off. This study provides further evidence that being physically active and including more intense activities (even if it's in the form of interval training) is critically important to staying thinner long-term. Resistance training is also a key to maintaining muscle mass and long-term body weight.

Results from the Why WAIT program are very similar to those reported by the NWCR. In fact, we always tell our participants at the end of the 12 weeks that the most helpful three bits of advice for maintaining weight loss over the long haul are the following:

1. EXERCISE
2. EXERCISE
3. EXERCISE

After the first year of follow-up, we found that the main characteristic of our former program participants who continued to maintain their weight or lose more is the duration of their daily exercise. People who continue to exercise for 250 to 300 minutes each week have been more successful in maintaining greater than 10 percent total weight loss beyond the program.

Lessons from the National Weight Control Registry

How do they keep it off? Most of the more than 10,000 people included in the National Weight Control Registry to date—that is, individuals who have maintained a minimum of 30 pounds of weight loss over at least one year—practice these key behaviors:

1. Eat (a healthy) breakfast every morning.

2. Watch their daily intake of calories.

3. Do high levels of exercise (average of 60 minutes daily).

4. Engage in daily self-monitoring of body weight. (This has been shown to be very important in catching weight regain early on.)

5. Most remain consistent with these behaviors across time (i.e., weekdays, weekends, holidays, vacations, etc.).

THE RIGHT FORMULA FOR SUSTAINED WEIGHT LOSS

Here's what we're proposing as the right formula for permanent weight loss:

Breakfast + Balanced Diet + Exercise + Weigh-ins = Successful Loser

Who knew that starting your day with a healthy breakfast was so important? It's one of the characteristics that almost all of the people included in the NWCR share, along with participating in regular physical activity, watching portion sizes, weighing in regularly, being consistent in their daily habits and continuing to eat a healthier diet overall.

The Diabetes Breakthrough program has already taught you a lot about how to prevent backsliding after you finish the initial 12-week program, as well as how to get back on track if you find yourself starting to regain weight.

Thanks to the Diabetes Breakthrough program, you now have the power, the tools, the ability and the desire to make your weight loss last.

Key Behaviors to Be a Successful "Loser" Yourself

1. Continue to count your daily calories.

2. Keep a logbook.

3. Set a weight loss goal.

4. Weigh in daily (by making it a part of your daily routine, like checking blood glucose).

5. Continue your current exercise plan at least five days per week for a total of at least 300 minutes a week (including three days with resistance training workouts).

6. Eat a healthy breakfast.

7. Maintain dietary consistency on all days, including weekends and holidays.

8. Be aware of portion control and a balanced plate.

YOUR EXERCISE PLAN FOR WEEK 11

You're continuing your target of doing 60 minutes of exercise almost every day of the week. Keep including aerobic, resistance and stretching activities, as well as combining them into interval training and other types of training, too. The importance of including varied exercises in your workouts can't be overstated. It's good for prevention of injuries and boredom. Also, the number of sets and reps during your resistance training can keep changing to give you progressive results. As you get stronger, you need to find new ways to challenge your muscles to burn more calories, which you can do by making them work harder. Try using a thicker resistance band, heavier free weights or more weight when using machines in the gym.

WEEK 11: DIABETES BREAKTHROUGH EXERCISE PLAN

DAY	AEROBIC	RESISTANCE	STRETCHING	TYPES OF EXERCISE
1	15 minutes	40 minutes	5 minutes	Aerobic, including interval training
2	55 minutes		5 minutes	Resistance, including superset training
3	15 minutes	40 minutes	5 minutes	(3 sets, 12 repetitions) Stretching
4				
5	55 minutes		5 minutes	
6	15 minutes	40 minutes	5 minutes	
7	55 minutes		5 minutes	
TOTAL TIME: 60 MINUTES				

THE DIFFERENCE BETWEEN LAPSE AND RELAPSE

Everyone has slips from time to time when working on changing long-standing behaviors. Some keys are to plan ahead to successfully manage future slips. You'll do well to adopt the health behaviors that are common to people who not only lose weight, but who are successful at keeping it off long-term. Having a clearly defined, written personal weight maintenance plan will help with staying on track after the program.

This week, we're going to discuss how behavioral lapses or slips can lead you to abandon your weight loss or diabetes self-care efforts and the strategies you will use to handle these slips in the future. Do you know what the difference is between a slip (lapse) and relapse? How would you define the difference?

Slips or lapses are to be expected; they're a natural part of learning to make long-term lifestyle changes. A slip is usually not a big deal, but if you react to it by returning to old negative thought patterns or by feeling guilty or ashamed, there's a good chance this single lapse will turn into a longer period of relapse. When such a scenario occurs, you could find yourself totally giving up on your plan and reverting back to old unhealthy behaviors.

The real key to maintaining weight loss is preventing relapse. By now, you have probably learned things about yourself that will help you in the future. By planning ahead for what you will do after the Diabetes Breakthrough program ends, you'll increase your likelihood of being successful at maintaining your weight loss and your diabetes improvements. Although maintaining weight loss can be challenging, it can definitely be done.

Lapse and Relapse

Lapses and slips are expected parts of any behavior change plan. This is a natural part of the process of learning to make long-term lifestyle changes. How you think about what happened is the key to preventing a relapse. The thoughts following a slip tend to be negative and self-defeating. The feelings of guilt, blame and self-defeat may lead to more overeating, feeling worse, more negative feelings and thoughts and more overeating. The single lapse or slip has now created a cycle of relapse.

The Bottom Line: Your reaction to the slip is what matters. The slip itself never really does much harm. The key is to engage in creative problem-solving after a slip so that you can see what led up to it, how to get yourself back on track and what you can learn from it.

Start thinking about what parts of the program you have found to be the most helpful and figure out ways to keep using them on your own as you move into phase two—the rest of your life after the program. For example, if frequent weigh-ins or keeping a logbook worked for you, hold on to these habits after the weekly program ends. One individual bought a 99-cent spiral notebook to log what he eats and does for exercise. It's small enough that it fits into his pants pocket and he keeps it with him all the time. You need to figure out what works for you and stick with it.

Day-Timer® and At-A-Glance® make planners that are designed to be a logbook and calendar specifically for people with diabetes and they are available online. Other companies also have similar products and online venues. In fact, you can find numerous online websites with tracking features and downloadable apps that work on both smartphones and tablets to track your food and exercise. Some examples include free apps like OnTrack Diabetes, Glucose Buddy and Diabetes IQ, as well as apps you can purchase such as LogFrog DB, iRecordit and Glooko Logbook.

Research has shown that simply weighing yourself regularly and frequently (and tracking changes in your weight) can be a helpful tool in weight loss management. Another successful program participant prints out a monthly calendar and tracks her weight changes daily by logging it on the calendar that hangs near her scale in the bathroom. However, this strategy doesn't work for everyone. If seeing a small fluctuation on the scale gets you into a cycle of negative thinking, weighing yourself daily may not be the best idea for you. Maybe weighing yourself once a week is enough. In either case, it's important to know when you are gaining weight so that you don't wake up one morning only to find that you're now 20 pounds heavier. Another thing that can really help you stay on track is having peers that are supportive of you and your new lifestyle.

Tips for Managing Lapses or Slips
- Analyze the situation and examine all the details to help you recognize and anticipate your high-risk situations the next time.
- Stay calm and talk back to negative thoughts with positive strategies.
- Renew your goals and review your progress.
- Take charge using problem-solving and your alternate activities list—that is, delay, delay, delay—until you outlast the urge the next time.
- Seek out support.
- Be wary of sabotage and misguided helpers.

IT'S OFF FOR GOOD
After completing the Why WAIT program several years ago, Velda is convinced that she holds all the cards now when it comes to keeping her weight under control. "The program convinced me that nutrition and exercise are the

keys to losing weight and to keeping it off," she says. "I guess I never took the exercise part seriously enough because it was easier just to eat more cottage cheese than to be active."

The program helped her permanently lose the weight that she had never succeeded in taking off and keeping off before. "Now I know what's next— good health for the rest of my life," she says with a big smile on her face. Are you smiling yet?

DIABETES BREAKTHROUGH WEEK 12

*Your Personal Weight Maintenance Plan and
Survival Tips for Down the Road*

You've reached the last formal week of the Diabetes Breakthrough program, which focuses on multiple areas. To see how far you've come, you'll weigh in again and retake the physical activity barriers quiz you did at the start of the program. If you still have barriers standing in your way, you'll set up some new SMART goals this week to help you deal with them. Finally, you'll find out the program's survival tips that you can use to manage your weight and keep your diabetes in check (or gone) for the rest of your life.

HEART ATTACK OR A HEALTHIER LIFE? YOUR CHOICE

At age 58, Richard was worried about having a heart attack or stroke because he knew the dangers of high blood glucose—they greatly increase his risk for cardiovascular disease. "My A1C values were up in the high 9's," he recalls. "After I spent two and a half weeks in critical care with sleep apnea and a mini-stroke, it was time to decide if I was going to be like my dad, who didn't live that long with type 2 diabetes—he died in his early 70's—or if I wanted to live." What choice do you think Richard made for himself?

WHY OLDER PEOPLE ARE INACTIVE

Many studies have addressed barriers to participation in regular physical activity over the years, but new research published in the *Journal of Geriatric Physical Therapy* recently shed some additional light on what keeps many older individuals less active. For starters, sedentary adults over 60 have much lower fitness expectations for being "active" and more overall barriers. In order to start exercising, they want someone to individually tailor an exercise program for them, they don't want to work out in gyms (they find them intimidating) and they are concerned that they'll slow others down if they join an exercise class.

Inactive older adults also want exercise to be purposeful and fun. Most important, most of these inactive individuals already perceive themselves as being active—maybe because they're more active than some of the older people around them—even if they're not really. If you want to be active, though, you'll need to develop strategies that allow you to overcome your barriers and the Diabetes Breakthrough program has hopefully already helped you develop them.

KEEP KNOCKING DOWN YOUR BARRIERS

Overcoming all the excuses you use to avoid making and sustaining lifestyle change is admittedly one of the hardest things you'll ever do, but it's certainly possible (and advisable). Taking a realistic look at your barriers to exercise, for example, can teach you which stumbling blocks to look out for. Learning more about how to control your cravings and urges and how to manage stress in more constructive ways will also help you stay on the path to sustained weight loss. It's up to you to plug in to the support and strategies that this program has presented you with to help you succeed in reversing your diabetes and managing your weight for better health.

Remember that "Barriers to Being Active Quiz" you completed the first week of the program? Now is the time to go back and take that quiz again—and pat yourself on the back for all the many ways that you have overcome so many of your barriers in the ensuing weeks. Take a hard look, though, at the areas where you could still improve and set some SMART goals to make strides in those areas, as well. We are confident you can overcome them all.

YOUR EXERCISE PLAN FOR WEEK 12

During this final week of the formal program, plan again on engaging in a variety of different types of exercise training. Your goal remains 60 minutes of daily exercise at least six days this week. Feel free to focus on doing more of the ones you love and even try some new aerobic activities or combinations of all different types. The key is to keep it fresh and enjoyable. Find a way to keep exercise as part of your new lifestyle. Remember that exercise is your new "medication" for controlling both your diabetes and your weight.

WEEK 12: DIABETES BREAKTHROUGH EXERCISE PLAN

DAY	AEROBIC	RESISTANCE	STRETCHING	TYPES OF EXERCISE
1	15 minutes	40 minutes	5 minutes	Aerobic, including interval training
2	55 minutes		5 minutes	Resistance, including superset training (3 sets, 12 repetitions)
3	15 minutes	40 minutes	5 minutes	Stretching
4				
5	55 minutes		5 minutes	
6	15 minutes	40 minutes	5 minutes	
7	55 minutes		5 minutes	

TOTAL TIME: 60 MINUTES

CREATE A PERSONAL WEIGHT MAINTENANCE PLAN

Now is the time to write out your weight maintenance plan—sort of like entering into a contract with yourself. Putting your plan in writing allows you to actually see what your goals are, rather than just keeping it all in your head, and will additionally help you stay focused on what you need to do to stay on track.

Make sure that your plans are well-defined, revisiting the use of SMART behavioral goals that we discussed at the start of this program. This is something for you to continue to work on because it's the basis of your plan for maintaining success. Think of this as a dynamic plan that will change as you change; you'll always be revising and adding to your goals. Make certain that your SMART goals are realistic and clearly defined. The following plan outline is adapted from an excellent book called *Cognitive-Behavioral Treatment of Obesity: A Clinician's Guide* by Z. Cooper, C. G. Fairburn and D. M. Hawker (Guilford Press, 2003).

Your Diabetes Breakthrough Weight Maintenance Plan

Why I don't want to regain weight:

_____

_____

_____

_____

New eating habits I plan to continue:

_____

_____

_____

_____

New exercise habits I plan to continue:

_____

_____

_____

_____

How I will know when I am slipping:

Example: Choose a frequency to weigh yourself and a weight regain range that will trigger you to start problem-solving or to seek out social support to continue.

Example: Choose a blood glucose range that will be a warning sign that things are slipping.

Example: How will you design your own logging system (how often, what to log, etc.)?

Example: Where will you keep your Diabetes Breakthrough logbook?

_____

_____

_____

_____

_____

_____

Remember: There's a difference between lapse and relapse.

Diabetes Breakthrough Survival Tips (for Down the Road)

1. Remember that calorie balance is most important, so be careful of your portions and if you want to eat more of one food, you need to eat less of another.

2. Vegetables are your friend. When in doubt, always reach for more nonstarchy vegetables or garden salad.

3. Sugar-free Jell-O® with a dollop of Cool Whip® can be a very satisfying treat.

4. You will have easier days and more difficult days; put the more difficult days behind you and keep moving forward.

5. Weigh yourself often and check your blood glucose as prescribed. As soon as you start to get off track with either weight or blood glucose, seek outside help.

6. EXERCISE, EXERCISE, EXERCISE.

7. Keep yourself away from food areas as best as you can, whether it is the kitchen or buffet tables.

continued

8. Plan ahead. This can't be emphasized enough. Don't try to fly by the seat of your pants when it comes to eating.

9. If there is a food you love, try to enjoy a small portion outside the home so it doesn't call to you from the refrigerator or cabinets.

10. You have accomplished amazing things in the past 12 weeks; it is now your time to continue your success and maintain it for a lifetime.

The Choice to Live—Long and Well

"I made the decision to live," Richard recalls. Although he enjoyed the heart-healthy diet, what Richard liked most about the Joslin Why WAIT program was the physical activity.

"Above all else, for me the exercise is important. I started out just doing treadmill. I had to get my heart in good shape to handle the rest and to work on my attitude. I didn't want to get there for quite a while. You have to want to."

He now controls his diabetes without insulin injections, which he used to give himself daily before he lost 60 pounds during the program and after. "It took deciding that I wanted to live and that I wanted to be healthy, too." Along with shedding his unhealthy lifestyle, he also shed his excess pounds—all because he made the right choice for his health.

PART II

THE
DIABETES
LIFE PLAN

DIABETES BREAKTHROUGH TO LASTING WEIGHT LOSS

We hope this program has been everything that you hoped it would be—for your weight loss, for your blood glucose control and for your personal growth. When it comes to maintaining not only your weight loss, but also your health, you will never stop learning things that can help you achieve your goals. This final chapter is a wrap-up of how far you've come (which you'll measure) and how to maintain these successes and gain new ones in the years to come.

IT'S ALL ABOUT MY FAMILY

In the end, for most people life is all about families and living life to the fullest with a healthy body. Diabetes can be a debilitating disease, which Sherry knew firsthand after seeing her grandmother suffer through heart attacks, strokes, amputations and other complications associated with it—and then Sherry was diagnosed with diabetes herself. At age 48, Sherry's experience with the Joslin Why WAIT program reinforced all that she knew she had to do to take care of herself. "I don't want to live the end of my life like my grandmother did," she states. "She couldn't feed herself and she couldn't even communicate with anyone after all her strokes. Her life was not worth living for the last six years she was alive." One thing Sherry knows for sure is that she wants her life story to progress differently. Is genetics her destiny? Or can she live her life with a better outcome? We'll let you know the answers to those questions shortly.

STOP DIABETES IN ITS TRACKS

There's no doubt that the Joslin Why WAIT program works and you should have achieved similar benchmarks from the Diabetes Breakthrough program that you've completed on your own. How did you do? In 12 weeks, Why WAIT participants lose almost 25 pounds and 3.6 inches from their waistlines. Their weight loss is steady, ranging from 1.2 to 2.5 pounds per week and they're losing bad belly fat to boot.

What about keeping it off? Unlike in other unproven programs, former Why WAIT participants are successful "losers," keeping most of the weight off for four years or more. Fifty percent of participants have successfully maintained all the weight they lost or continued to lose weight for four years (around 24 pounds after that time, or about 9.5 percent), while retaining most of their muscle mass. In fact, the average weight loss for all Why WAIT participants after four years, including those who gained some weight back, is still an astounding 6.3 percent. Most important, they have cut their medication doses by about 50 percent and experienced a tremendous improvement in their quality of life. This program is your best chance to stop diabetes progression in its tracks.

ADOPT LIFELONG LIFESTYLE HABITS

By now, you've hopefully realized that all of the lifestyle changes you've made to lose weight and reverse your diabetes are more than temporary habits. The difference between a diet and a lifestyle is that one is a short-lived sprint and the other involves a commitment to an ongoing process. Diabetes is a chronic condition, so it requires this kind of long-term commitment. Weight struggles are also long-term and also require continuous work.

You assuredly won't be dieting forever, but you will be following a dietary plan for the rest of your life. Remember, a diet is a reduced-calorie intake followed temporarily to lose weight, but a dietary plan is a more permanent change in your eating habits that will allow you to keep the weight off. You should also plan on continuing to exercise for 60 minutes per day, six days per week, whenever possible and you understand why you need to adopt activities that you can do for the rest of your life, such as brisk walking, intervals and resistance training to maintain your muscle mass. As Dr. Hamdy always says, "The best three ways to help maintain long-term weight loss are exercise, exercise and exercise!"

EQUIPPED FOR THE REST OF YOUR LIFE

Now that you've finished this 12-week program, you've never been better equipped to take your life—and your body weight—into your own hands for the rest of your life. You're equipped with tools that you can use for the rest of your life that are guaranteed to help you make the journey with less body fat than ever before. What's more, you're armed with the know-how to keep the weight off and your diabetes in check (or gone) for the rest of your life.

If you've eliminated your diabetes medications (or hope to reduce them further), you can stay off of them if you maintain the healthy lifestyle changes that you've learned and practiced for the past three months. Your body is your temple and you've already shown that you're capable of caring for it in ways that you never thought possible before. Go forward with confidence that your best years are yet to come.

MEASURE YOURSELF AGAIN AND MOVE ON TO THE REST OF YOUR LIFE

It's always good to have an ending place, too, to see when you've improved and how much. Now is the time to repeat the measurements you took at the start of this program to see just how far you've already come. Seeing your progress will allow you to set new SMART goals for the weeks, months and years of your life to come. Don't forget to congratulate yourself on any improvements.

> **Weigh in:** Weigh yourself on a scale at the same time of day under similar circumstances (e.g., after your morning shower, without clothes or with the same minimal clothing on and before eating breakfast) as you did in Week 1. How do you feel about how far you've come?

Measure up: Use a tape measure to remeasure your waist, your hips and anywhere else you chose to measure in Week 1. If you've lost even an inch, you have succeeded. (Remeasure your body fat, too, if you did that 12 weeks ago.)

Pick a pair: Put on those pants you picked during Week 1. How do they fit? If they're looser, you're a "loser."

Walk a bit: Use the same route or treadmill to do another six-minute walk test. Can you go farther now? We'd be shocked if you can't. Hopefully, you also feel more energetic overall, healthier, stronger and more flexible, as well.

ACTIVE, EATING AND HEALTHY FOR LIFE

There are three main elements in this program that you need to always keep in mind: medication change and blood glucose checks, improvements to your meal plan and an ongoing exercise routine. In order to keep these three pieces going, you need to do a lot of active monitoring to catch potential wobble points early and give yourself opportunities to regroup. Given that these are long-range strategies, the monitoring needs to remain a long-term tool that you use.

Think about what it feels like to be living in your body now versus 12 weeks ago. What feels better? Remember what the feeling of "wellness" is like. You are in your body right now and changes are still ongoing. While some people are looking to completely transform themselves, doing that may not be possible or even necessary. However, maintaining the improvements you have already achieved is critical. If you can maintain the heightened sense of wellness you have right now—including improved fitness, weight loss and blood glucose management—then you've already achieved wellness. Set your current weight as your new maximum and work to keep yourself below it over the long haul.

10 Steps for Maintaining Success

1. Set realistic, achievable SMART goals and expectations for yourself, for your diabetes control, weight loss and exercise. Don't try to do everything at once. Start new changes gradually. Diabetes is a chronic disease, so your goals and expectations need to be maintainable and sustainable.

2. Plan ahead. What will make it easier for you to stick to a meal plan and exercise plan? Think of this as a life commitment to your health and fitness. Build in time for exercise. Give yourself variety in your exercise and meal plan so that you don't get bored or feel deprived.

3. Focus on positive rewards for yourself rather than negative consequences. Self-criticism and fear of diabetes complications are not good motivators for success. Think of ways to reward yourself and praise yourself for positive changes, rather than berate yourself for slips.

4. Learn from what has worked for you in the past and do it again. Even if it only worked for brief periods of time, build on your small experiences of success.

5. Decide that you and your health are worth the effort it will take to make these changes. This is a tough one, because weight, fitness and self-worth in our culture are often measured in direct opposition to each other. (The more you weigh, the worse you feel about yourself and the less you may feel you are worth the effort.)

6. Find the support you need: family, friends, spouses, coworkers, join clubs or support groups. Be aware of misguided helping and the "diabetes police."

7. Create a supportive medical team: primary care doctor, endocrinologist, nutritionist, nurse educator, exercise physiologist, mental health practitioner. Make sure that you all share the same goals and that they are on your side. Remember: you are the most important player on this team.

8. Use assertiveness when you need it. This is especially important when you feel you are surrounded by unwanted help or undue

continued

scrutiny by others. Friends and loved ones want to help, but they may need clear communication from you about how to help and what you need from them.

9. Keep track of your progress and slips on a daily basis. Research shows that people who routinely monitor their progress are more likely to maintain weight loss and fitness goals. Remember that slips are normal and expectable.

10. Plan for prevention during high-risk situations where you are likely to slip. The more you monitor yourself, the more you'll learn about what times are the riskiest for you and how to creatively come up with solutions to avoid slipping.

YOUR EXERCISE PLAN FOR WEEK 13 AND BEYOND (THE REST OF YOUR LIFE)

The world is your oyster when it comes to your lifetime exercise plan. Your main goal is to keep on exercising nearly every day for the rest of your life. That may sound daunting, but it really doesn't have to be. Mix it up, make it fun, do it with others and keep yourself injury-free by varying your routines. The most important point is just do something. Easy days, harder workouts, different types of activities—all of these are fine in the realm of a lifelong exercise plan. Just revisit your barriers occasionally and set new SMART goals to continue to overcome them. Remember to credit all your daily steps toward your exercise goals. When there's a will, there's a way.

LIFETIME PLAN: DIABETES BREAKTHROUGH EXERCISE PLAN

DAY	AEROBIC	RESISTANCE	STRETCHING	TYPES OF EXERCISE
1	15 minutes	40 minutes	5 minutes	All types
2	55 minutes		5 minutes	
3	15 minutes	40 minutes	5 minutes	

4				All types
5	55 minutes		5 minutes	
6	15 minutes	40 minutes	5 minutes	
7	55 minutes		5 minutes	
TOTAL TIME: 60 MINUTES				

TRAINING OPTIONS TO KEEP WEIGHT OFF FOR GOOD

To mix things up and keep your training fresh, try a combination of cross, interval and superset training (3 sets, 12 reps), along with stretching. Come up with some of your own routines to use, as well as the following:

Combo Workout #1

1. 10 minutes interval training
2. Rowing and chest press
3. 3 minutes aerobic/30 seconds intervals
4. Biceps curls and triceps press
5. 3 minutes aerobic/30 seconds intervals
6. Side-to-side steps (walking to right and left) and lat pull down
7. 3 minutes aerobic/30 seconds intervals
8. Upright rowing and squat
9. 3 minutes aerobic/30 seconds intervals
10. Heel raises and shoulder press
11. 3 minutes aerobic/30 seconds intervals
12. Trunk twist (to one side and then other side)
13. 3 minutes aerobic/30 seconds intervals
14. Stretching

Combo Workout #2

1. 10 minutes interval training
2. Front raises and squat
3. 3 minutes aerobic/30 seconds intervals

4. Heel raises and shoulder press
5. 3 minutes aerobic/30 seconds intervals
6. Upright row and triceps press
7. 3 minutes aerobic/30 seconds intervals
8. Trunk twist (to one side and then other side)
9. 3 minutes aerobic/30 seconds intervals
10. Biceps curls and chest press
11. 3 minutes aerobic/30 seconds intervals
12. Side-to-side steps and lat pull down
13. 3 minutes aerobic/30 seconds intervals
14. Stretching

Combo Workout #3

1. 30 minutes interval training
2. Heel raises and squat
3. Rowing and side-to-side steps
4. Lat pull down and upright row
5. Triceps press and biceps curls
6. Chest press and heel raises
7. Alternate front arm raise and lunge step backward
8. Plank or modified plank and bridging with or without straight leg raises
9. Stretching

HOW MUCH EXERCISE IS ENOUGH?

To lose weight, it is generally recommended that you get 60 minutes of exercise at least six or seven days per week. To maintain weight loss, you will likely need to continue doing a similar amount of exercise. However, all activity during the day counts toward that total, not just your planned activities. You can get your total time in by doing several bouts throughout the day: for example, you could do two 15-minute bouts of walking or biking during the day and then 30 minutes of resistance training with bands or use the gym in the evening. Doing more vigorous activities and intervals also burns off more calories in less time.

All of your daily steps and other movement count toward this goal as well—so move more all day long. Even if you get up from your desk and walk around for five minutes at the end of every hour during an eight-hour day, you'll burn over an extra 130 calories a day just from doing that. Sometimes that little extra expenditure is all it takes to keep the weight off.

Strategies to Keep the Weight Off
- Continue to count calories.
- Set a weight loss goal.
- Keep a daily or weekly logbook.
- Weigh in daily (i.e., make it a routine).
- Continue contact with your weight loss support system on a weekly basis.
- If you regain more than two pounds, take some time to revisit your diet and exercise habits to see what you need to do to get back on track.
- Continue your current exercise plan at least six days per week for 60 minutes and include three days a week of resistance training as part of that total.
- Eat a healthy breakfast.
- Maintain dietary consistency, including on weekends and holidays.
- Be aware of portion control and a balanced plate.
- Don't forget to exercise, exercise, exercise.

COUNT YOUR DAILY STEPS

All participants in the Why WAIT program are given pedometers (step counters). It is used as a motivational tool to increase your activity level. If you don't already have a pedometer to track your daily steps, you can easily pick up an inexpensive one that will help you get a better feel for your daily activity. If you can't get a pedometer, however, don't despair. You can always estimate the step equivalents of many of the activities that you do during the day and it's possible to simply estimate your steps instead.

Pedometers work for many people as a motivational tool; however, if you have a major joint or foot problem that limits your walking and using a stationary cycling or other seated activity is your main aerobic exercise, don't feel obligated to start walking to count steps. It may exacerbate your medical problem and could lead to more barriers.

Get the Most Out of Your Pedometer

- Pedometers only count steps during walking, jogging, running, etc., but they won't count steps during cycling, rowing, upper body exercise, swimming and other activities. Estimate these to get credit for them using the step equivalent table below.

- For most adults, 2,000 steps is the equivalent of about one mile of walking, but the recorded steps can be affected by stride length, pedometer accuracy and other factors.

- Go for simplicity, but accuracy, in a pedometer. They're most accurate in counting steps, less accurate in calculating distance walked and even less accurate at estimating caloric expenditure. You don't need all the special features, just the step count.

- Most pedometers are fairly accurate step counters at speeds of 2.5 mph and above.

- Attach them to a firm waistband in an upright position and placed to the side (directly in line with one of your knees; loose waistbands typically underestimate steps).

- If you have a larger abdomen, place the pedometer at the small of your back, or alternately use one that works when placed in a pocket or other location.

- To test your pedometer's accuracy, position it on your belt or waistband in line with one knee on either side and reset its count to zero. Walk 20 steps at a typical walking pace—it should record between 18 and 22 steps. If it repeatedly fails this test, look into getting another type.

- Recommended brands include most Omron®, Accusplit® and Yamax® models.

CALCULATE YOUR DAILY STEPS AND ADD 500 MORE

Simply taking more daily steps can help improve your diabetes, control your weight, cholesterol and blood pressure and make you feel better. Start walking and count your daily number of steps by wearing a pedometer to determine your baseline. Then increase the number of steps you take and watch how your blood glucose control improves.

Follow these steps to calculate your average daily number to have a baseline number:

STEP 1: Use a pedometer to count the number of steps you take in seven days and record in the table below. Remember to reset your pedometer every morning.

	MON	TUES	WED	THURS	FRI	SAT	SUN	TOTAL
STEPS								

STEP 2: Add up all the steps you took in seven days. Divide it by seven to get the average number of steps you take in a day.

Total number of steps in seven days:
_____ ÷ 7 = _____ daily average steps.

For example: number of steps in seven days is
22,400 ÷ 7 = 3,200 daily average steps.

STEP 3: Add 500 steps to your daily average steps every two weeks. From the last example, your daily average steps number is 3,200. Your goal should be to add 500 steps each day for the next two weeks and record it in your logbook. For best results, calculate your new daily average number of steps every two weeks and try to add 500 to that amount.

If you don't have access to a pedometer, it's also possible to estimate the number of daily steps based on any activities that you do. Some typical equivalent step values follow.

STEPS EQUIVALENTS FOR VARIOUS PHYSICAL ACTIVITIES

ACTIVITY	STEPS IN 1 MINUTE	STEPS IN 15 MINUTES	STEPS IN 30 MINUTES
Aerobic dance	197	2,955	5,910
Ballroom dancing, slow to fast	91–167	1,365–2,505	2,730–5,010
Bowling	91	1,365	2,730
Canoeing	106	1,590	3,180
Circuit training	242	3,630	7,260
Climbing, rock or mountain	273	4,095	8,190
Gardening	121	1,815	3,630
Golf	136	2,040	4,080
Gymnastics	121	1,815	3,630
Hiking	182	2,730	5,460
Jogging	212	3,180	6,360
Jogging on minitrampoline	136	2,040	4,080
Martial arts	303	4,545	9,090
Running, 5–8 mph	242–409	3,630–6,135	7,260–12,270
Shopping	70	1,050	2,100
Stationary cycling, moderate to vigorous	212–318	3,180–4,770	6,360–9,540
Step aerobics	273	4,095	8,190
Swimming laps, moderate to vigorous	212–303	3,180–4,545	6,360–9,090
Swimming leisurely	182	2,730	5,460
Water aerobics	121	1,815	3,630
Water jogging	242	3,630	7,260
Weight lifting, moderate to vigorous	121–182	1,815–2,730	3,630–5,460
Yoga and stretching	76	1,140	2,280

DON'T LET THIS BE YOU

Here's an example of what to try to avoid: We had an individual in the Joslin Why WAIT program who felt that "all of a sudden," he regained 11 pounds. Well, this clearly did not happen overnight. What changed?

When we asked him what happened, he replied, "I'm done—with everything." What he meant was he was no longer weighing himself daily, keeping a food or blood glucose record, or exercising regularly and he had reverted back to his old food choices. That's what changed. Your job is to use everything you've learned in this program to keep that from happening to you.

If you should fall off the wagon for any reason (e.g., illness, vacation, emotional upset), get yourself back on track as soon as possible using familiar principles like SMART goal-setting, analyzing your slips and talking yourself out of your negative thinking. To make sure a complete relapse gets avoided and slips get nipped in the bud, do your best to maintain everything you have learned and achieved in this program.

CONQUER OR SUFFER

What made Sherry join the Joslin Why WAIT program after her diabetes diagnosis? She simply made a decision to conquer her diabetes instead of succumbing to it or its potential health complications.

She says, "This program has made such a difference in my life and in the lives of those who love me and are concerned about my health. I'm now able to spend better quality time with my family and friends and feel good." For her, that's what matters the most—especially when she has decades more to go while living a long and healthy life.

Your success depends on your actions.

BREAKFAST MENU CHOICES

Choose one selection from each list (carbohydrate and protein).

Carbohydrate

1. ¾ cup whole grain cereal (milk) (>5 gm fiber)
2. 2 slices whole grain bread
3. 1 whole wheat English muffin
4. 1 small (2 ounces) whole wheat bagel
5. 2 whole wheat waffles and ¼ cup sugar-free syrup
6. ½ cup cooked oatmeal or 1 packet
7. 6 ounces light yogurt and 1 fruit serving
8. ½ whole wheat English muffin or 1 slice whole wheat toast and 1 fruit serving
9. 1 slice whole wheat toast and 6 ounces light yogurt
10. ¼ cup cooked oatmeal and 6 ounces light yogurt
11. ¼ cup cooked oatmeal and 1 fruit serving

Protein

1. 1 low-fat chicken sausage and 1 tablespoon light, trans fat–free spread
2. 1 egg or ¼ cup egg substitute and 1 tablespoon light, trans fat–free spread
3. 2 eggs or ½ cup egg substitute and 1 slice light cheese
4. 2 slices Canadian bacon and 1 tablespoon light, trans fat–free spread
5. 1 ounce nuts (¼ cup)
6. 1½ tablespoons peanut butter

7. ¾ cup low-fat cottage cheese

8. 2 tablespoons light cream cheese and 1 low-fat chicken sausage or 2 slices Canadian bacon or 1 egg (¼ cup egg substitute)

9. 2 slices light cheese or 2 slices 2% milk cheese and 1 tablespoon light, trans fat–free spread

Total Calories per breakfast = approximately 300

Nutrition Facts: All Calorie Plans
AVERAGES FOR BREAKFAST CHOICES

TOTAL CALORIES: 300

	Grams	Calories	% Calories
CARBS	30-34	120-136	40-45
PROTEIN	15-22	60-88	20-30
FAT	10-12	90-108	30-35

Breakfast Menu Examples

1. ½ cup dry oatmeal or 1 oatmeal packet plus 1½ tablespoons peanut butter or 3 tablespoons chopped nuts

2. 1 whole wheat English muffin or 2 slices whole wheat toast (avg. 80 calories per slice) or 1 small whole wheat bagel (2 ounces) with 1½ tablespoons peanut butter

3. 1 whole wheat English muffin or 2 slices whole wheat toast (avg. 80 calories per slice) or 1 small whole wheat bagel (2 ounces) with 1 cup low-fat cottage cheese

4. 1 whole wheat English muffin or 2 slices whole wheat toast (avg. 80 calories per slice) or 1 small whole wheat bagel (2 ounces) with 1 egg or ½ cup egg beaters and 1 slice low-fat/light cheese and 1 teaspoon trans fat–free spread such as Smart Balance® or 2 teaspoons light trans fat–free spread such as Smart Balance Light®

5. 2 whole wheat waffles with ¼ cup sugar-free syrup and 2 teaspoons light spread or 1 teaspoon regular spread and 1 low-fat chicken sausage or 2 ounces Canadian bacon

6. 6 ounces light or plain yogurt with 1 fruit serving and 3 tablespoons chopped nuts

7. 1 slice whole wheat toast with 1½ tablespoons peanut butter and ½ medium-to-large banana

8. Diabetes-friendly meal replacement shake: Ultra Glucose Control®, Boost Glucose Control®, Boost Calorie Smart® or Glucerna Hunger Smart® with 1 tablespoon nuts and 1 fruit serving

LUNCH MENU EXCHANGES
Protein Selections
Goal: approximately 25 grams or 3.5 ounces protein per lunch
1 ounce = 7 grams protein

1-ounce servings:
- Tuna—¼ cup
- Lean roast beef—weigh, typical 1 deli slice
- Lean turkey—weigh, typical 1 deli slice
- Low sodium ham—weigh, typical 1 deli slice
- Chicken—weigh
- Low-fat cottage cheese—¼ cup
- Low-fat cheese slices—1 slice
- Nuts—¼ cup or 4 tablespoons
- Peanut butter—1½ tablespoons
- Egg—1 egg

Carbohydrate-containing protein sources
(need to count as both protein and carb)
- Beans—½ cup (15 grams carb)
- Hummus—⅓ cup (7 grams carb)
- Milk—1 cup/8 ounces (12 grams carb)
- Yogurt—3 ounces plain Greek-style yogurt,
  4 ounces plain, 6 ounces light (12 grams carb)

Other products: veggie burgers, mixed foods such as soups and chili. Read the label for protein grams. Be aware that they may also contain carbohydrates.

Carbohydrate Selections
Goal: 30 grams carb per lunch
1 carb serving = 15 grams carb unless otherwise noted

Milk products = 12 grams carb

1 ounce bread product tends to be 15 grams carb, depending on fiber content

Remember to subtract fiber from total carbohydrates to reach 30 grams (excluding fiber)
- Whole wheat pita—1 ounce, approximately 4" diameter; read label as they vary
- Whole wheat tortilla/wrap—1 ounce, approximately 6–8" diameter; read label as they vary
- Whole wheat bread—1 ounce slice; read label as they vary
- Fruit—see fruit list for serving size
- Whole grain crackers—read label as they vary

Protein-containing carb sources (need to count as both protein and carb)
- Yogurt—4 ounces plain, 6 ounces light
- Milk—1 cup/8 ounces
- Beans—½ cup

Fat Selections
Goal: approximately 12 grams fat per lunch
1 serving = 5 grams fat

Typically only add 1 fat serving per lunch since the protein options usually contain fat, as well. If the proteins are very low in fat, add 2 fat servings.
- Guacamole—2 tablespoons
- Light sour cream—2 tablespoons
- Light mayonnaise—1 tablespoon
- Light salad dressing—2 tablespoons
- Light trans fat–free spread—1 tablespoon
- Regular trans fat–free spread—½ tablespoon
- Oil—1 teaspoon

Total Calories per lunch = approximately 350–400

Nutrition Facts: All Calorie Plans
AVERAGES FOR LUNCH CHOICES

TOTAL CALORIES: 350–400

	Grams	Calories	% Calories
CARBS	35–39	140–157	40–45
PROTEIN	17–26	70–105	20–30
FAT	12–14	105–122	30–35

Adapted from Joslin Diabetes Center Why WAIT program materials.
Copyright © 2012 by Joslin Diabetes Center (www.joslin.org). All rights reserved.

12 LUNCH RECIPES (1 SERVING EACH)

TUNA SANDWICH ON WHOLE WHEAT PITA WITH BLACK BEAN SOUP

Ingredients:

2 ounces canned tuna,
drained of water

1 tablespoon light mayonnaise

2 tablespoons diced celery

1 small whole wheat pita

1 tablespoon dry-roasted,
unsalted almonds

1 cup black bean soup

Mix tuna, mayonnaise and celery together and serve in pita with almonds and black bean soup on the side.

ROAST BEEF SANDWICH ON WHOLE WHEAT PITA WITH HUMMUS AND CARROTS

Ingredients:

3 ounces low-sodium, lean roast beef

1 slice red onion

1 lettuce leaf

1 small whole wheat pita

¾ cup carrots

⅓ cup hummus

Make sandwich with roast beef, onion and lettuce on whole wheat pita and serve carrots and hummus on the side.

CHICKEN NOODLE SOUP WITH PEANUT BUTTER AND CRACKERS

Ingredients:

1 cup low-sodium chicken noodle soup

1½ tablespoons peanut butter

8 Kashi TLC crackers

Serve soup with peanut butter and crackers on the side.

BEAN AND CHICKEN BURRITO WITH SIDE SALAD

Ingredients:

½ cup canned black beans

3 tablespoons guacamole

3 ounces diced grilled chicken breast

1 whole wheat tortilla (approximately 70 calories)

1 cup mixed greens salad

1 tablespoon balsamic or red wine vinegar

Mix beans, guacamole and chicken and put into tortilla. Heat in microwave for one minute. Serve with side salad.

SALAD WITH WALNUTS AND CRANBERRIES AND SIDE OF YOGURT

Ingredients:

¼ cup chopped, unsalted walnuts

2 tablespoons dried cranberries

3 cups garden salad

1 tablespoon balsamic vinegar

4 ounces light yogurt

Mix walnuts and cranberries together on top of salad with dressing and have yogurt on the side.

ENGLISH MUFFIN PIZZA

Ingredients:

¼ cup canned pizza sauce

1 whole wheat English muffin

¼ cup part skim mozzarella cheese

3 ounces low-fat chicken sausage

2 slices tomato

4 strips fresh green pepper

Spread pizza sauce on English muffin halves and add cheese, chicken sausage and vegetables. Bake in oven at 350°F for 10–12 minutes.

COTTAGE CHEESE WITH FRUIT AND TOAST WITH PEANUT BUTTER

Ingredients:

¾ cup low-fat cottage cheese

6 ounces fruit (approximately 1 cup)

1 slice whole wheat, light bread

1 tablespoon peanut butter

Mix fruit with cottage cheese and serve with peanut butter toast.

GREEK SALAD

Ingredients:

3 cups garden salad

¼ cup crumbled feta cheese

5 black olives

¼ cup whole wheat croutons

2 tablespoons Greek dressing

4 ounces fresh pear

Mix ingredients for salad together and add dressing. Serve with pear on the side.

CHEF SALAD

Ingredients:

3 cups garden salad

1 hard-boiled egg

1 slice (1 ounce) low-sodium ham

1 slice (1 ounce) low-sodium turkey

2 tablespoons light ranch dressing

5 ounces apple

Mix ingredients for salad together and add dressing. Serve with apple on the side or dice apple into salad.

VEGETARIAN BURGER WITH SIDE SALAD

Ingredients:

1 vegetarian burger patty

1 slice light cheddar cheese

2 slices whole wheat, light bread

½ tablespoon light
Thousand Island dressing

1 cup garden salad

1 tablespoon balsamic
or red wine vinegar

Microwave vegetarian burger for one and a half minutes then melt cheese on vegetarian burger in the microwave. Place vegetarian burger in between slices of bread and add dressing to burger. Serve with side garden salad sprinkled with vinegar.

TURKEY AND AVOCADO WRAP WITH APPLE

Ingredients:

3 ounces low-sodium turkey breast

2 lettuce leaves

1 slice medium tomato

1 tablespoon light mayonnaise

¼ sliced avocado

1 whole wheat tortilla (approximately
70 calories)

4 ounces apple

Place turkey, lettuce, tomato, mayonnaise and avocado in wrap and serve with apple on the side.

CHICKEN SALAD SANDWICH WITH SIDE OF SNOW PEAS

Ingredients:

3 ounces diced grilled chicken

1½ tablespoons light mayonnaise

2 tablespoons chopped red onion

⅛ teaspoon ground dill weed

⅛ teaspoon lemon juice

2 teaspoons chopped walnuts

2 slices whole wheat, light bread

1 cup snow peas

Mix together all the ingredients except the snow peas and place between two slices of whole wheat bread. Serve with snow peas on the side or side garden salad with vinegar if desired.

The total calories in the dinner meal vary the most based on which menu you are following: 1200, 1500 or 1800. Also refer to the lists given for Week 1 for food options (vegetable, fat, fruit and snack servings) and serving sizes, especially when filling one-third to one-half of your plate with vegetables.

Protein Selections
Goal: 6–8 ounces raw weight
1 ounce = 7 grams protein
Meat, poultry and fish cook down 1 ounce.

1-ounce servings:
- Tuna—¼ cup
- Meat—weigh
- Poultry—weigh
- Fish—weigh
- Low-fat cottage cheese—¼ cup
- Low-fat cheese slices—1 slice
- Nuts—¼ cup or 4 tablespoons
- Peanut butter—1½ tablespoons
- Egg—1 egg

Carbohydrate-containing protein sources
(need to count as both protein and carb)
- Beans—½ cup (15 grams carb)
- Hummus—⅓ cup (7 grams carb)
- Milk—1 cup/8 ounces (12 grams carb)
- Yogurt—3 ounces plain Greek-style yogurt, 4 ounces plain, 6 ounces light (12 grams carb)

Other products: veggie burgers, mixed foods such as soups and chili. Read the label for protein grams. Be aware that they may also contain carbohydrates.

Carbohydrate Selections
Goal: 45–75 grams carb per dinner, depending on meal plan
1 carb serving = 15 grams carb unless otherwise noted

Milk products = 12 grams carb

1 ounce bread product tends to be 15 grams carb, depending on fiber content

Remember to subtract fiber from total carbohydrates to reach 45–75 grams (excluding fiber)
- Brown rice—⅓ cup
- Whole wheat pasta—⅓ cup
- Potato—3 ounces (weigh)
- Sweet potato—2 ounces (weigh)
- Butternut squash—1 cup
- Corn—½ cup
- Peas—½ cup
- Whole wheat pita—1 ounce, approximately 4" diameter; read label as they vary
- Whole wheat tortilla/wrap—1 ounce, approximately 6–8" diameter; read label as they vary
- Whole wheat bread—1 ounce slice; read label as they vary
- Fruit—see fruit list for serving size
- Whole grain crackers—read label as they vary

Protein-containing carb sources (need to count as both protein and carb)
- Yogurt—4 ounces plain, 6 ounces light
- Milk—1 cup/8 ounces
- Beans—½ cup

Fat Selections
Goal: approximately 12 grams fat per dinner
1 serving = 5 grams fat

Typically only add 1 fat serving per dinner since the protein options usually contain fat, as well. If the proteins are very low in fat, add 2 fat servings.

- Guacamole—2 tablespoons
- Light sour cream—2 tablespoons
- Light mayonnaise—1 tablespoon
- Light salad dressing—2 tablespoons
- Light trans fat–free spread—1 tablespoon
- Regular trans fat–free spread—½ tablespoon
- Oil—1 teaspoon

Total Calories per dinner = approximately 500–700, depending on meal plan

Nutrition Facts: 1200-Calorie Plan

AVERAGES FOR DINNER CHOICES

TOTAL CALORIES: 500

	Grams	Calories	% Calories
CARBS	50–56	200–224	40–45
PROTEIN	25–37	100–150	20–30
FAT	17–19	153–171	30–35

Nutrition Facts: 1500-Calorie Plan

AVERAGES FOR DINNER CHOICES

TOTAL CALORIES: 600

	Grams	Calories	% Calories
CARBS	60–67	240–268	40–45
PROTEIN	30–45	120–180	20–30
FAT	20–23	180–207	30–35

Nutrition Facts: 1800-Calorie Plan
AVERAGES FOR DINNER CHOICES

TOTAL CALORIES: 700

	Grams	Calories	% Calories
CARBS	70–79	280–316	40–45
PROTEIN	35–52.5	140–210	20–30
FAT	23–41	207–369	30–35

12 DINNER RECIPES (1 SERVING EACH)

When cooking, keep in mind that these recipes are intended to be a single serving only (so if you are cooking for more than one or making extra servings for another day, increase the amounts accordingly). Each recipe varies slightly based on the calorie menu plan you are following (1200, 1500 or 1800) and differences for each recipe are included based on those plans in the list of ingredients for each serving. All meals follow the proven Joslin Why WAIT diet plan (carbohydrates 40–45 percent of total calories, protein 20–30 percent and fat 30–35 percent). They closely approximate the recommended calorie intake for dinner on each of the three plans (500, 600 and 700 calories, respectively). Make use of your measuring cups and spoons and kitchen scales to help you get the portion sizes as close as possible to what is intended.

MEDITERRANEAN COD

Ingredients:

2 ripe Roma tomatoes

2 tablespoons fresh green onion

2 large canned black olives without pits

4 fresh basil leaves

½ teaspoon garlic powder

2 teaspoons olive oil

2–3 tablespoons lemon juice

1 tablespoon balsamic vinegar

Black pepper to taste

7 ounces raw cod fillet for 1200; 8 ounces for 1500; 10 ounces for 1800

¾ cup whole wheat pasta (cooked portion) for 1200; 1 cup for 1500;
1¼ cups for 1800

½ cup light tomato-and-basil pasta sauce for 1200; ⅔ cup for 1500; ¾ cup for 1800

¼ pound (1 cup) of chopped fresh spinach

2 chopped garlic cloves

Cooking spray

Preheat oven to 425°F. Prepare a medium saucepan with 1 quart of water to boil. Wash and chop tomato, green onion, olives and fresh basil.

In a small bowl, combine chopped tomato, green onion, olives, basil, garlic powder, olive oil, half of the lemon juice, vinegar and black pepper to taste.

Lightly coat a shallow baking dish with nonstick cooking spray.

Rinse and pat dry the fish with a paper towel and season with black pepper. Place fish in prepared baking dish. Drizzle fish with remaining lemon juice and top with the tomato mixture.

Bake until just cooked through, approximately 10 to 12 minutes or until fish flakes easily with a fork.

While fish is cooking, prepare pasta and spinach. Boil pasta in a medium saucepan until tender; drain well and top with heated pasta sauce before serving. Sauté spinach with 2 cloves of chopped garlic in skillet with nonstick cooking spray until spinach wilts.

Nutrition Facts

DINNER 1: MEDITERRANEAN COD

PLAN	CALORIES	CARBS	PROTEIN	FAT	FIBER	SODIUM
1200	500	57	44	13	12	660
1500	630	69	51	18	14	810
1800	720	81	62	18	16	900

SALSA CHICKEN

Ingredients:

⅔ cup cooked whole wheat pasta for 1200; 1 cup for 1500; 1⅓ cups for 1800

1½ teaspoons extra virgin olive oil

1 minced garlic clove

6½ ounces raw skinless chicken breast for 1200; 7 ounces for 1500; 8 ounces for 1800

3 tablespoons salsa for 1200 and 1500; 4 teaspoons for 1800

2 teaspoons water

1 tablespoon natural seedless raisins

¼ teaspoon ground cumin

¼ teaspoon ground cinnamon

1 cup chopped raw carrots

1 teaspoon trans fat–free spread

Boil pasta in a medium saucepan and cook according to package directions.

Heat oil in a medium skillet over medium-high heat until hot. Add garlic to skillet; cook and stir 30 seconds. Add chicken and cook 4 to 5 minutes or until browned, turning once.

In a small bowl, combine salsa, water, raisins, cumin and ⅛ teaspoon of cinnamon; mix well.

Add mixture to chicken in skillet and stir. Reduce heat to medium; cover and cook 20 minutes or until chicken is no longer pink inside and juices run clear, stirring occasionally.

Steam carrots in microwave or on the stovetop until crisp-tender.

Add trans fat–free spread and remaining ⅛ teaspoon of cinnamon on carrots.

Serve salsa chicken with carrots on the side.

Nutrition Facts

DINNER 2: SALSA CHICKEN

PLAN	CALORIES	CARBS	PROTEIN	FAT	FIBER	SODIUM
1200	510	49	47	14	8	560
1500	570	62	51	14	10	540
1800	660	75	60	15	11	670

STEAK WITH ZUCCHINI

Ingredients:

⅓ medium zucchini squash

5–6 white mushrooms

½ medium onion

5 ounces raw beef, flank steak, London broil for 1200; 6.5 ounces for 1500; 7.5 ounces for 1800

¼ teaspoon Mrs. Dash steak seasoning

3 tablespoons balsamic vinegar

1 teaspoon olive oil

6 ounces red potato for 1200; 7 ounces for 1500; 9 ounces for 1800

2 tablespoons light sour cream

Chop zucchini into ½" chunks. Halve mushrooms and chop onion into ½" chunks.

Sprinkle steak with Mrs. Dash steak seasoning.

Arrange vegetables and steak in a large baking dish.

Mix balsamic vinegar and olive oil for dressing. Add dressing to vegetables and steak, turn and toss until well coated. Cover and let stand at room temperature for 20 minutes.

Preheat an outdoor grill or the broiler.

Prepare potato by washing and piercing with a fork several times; microwave on high until tender, turning once halfway through cooking time (this may take 5–10 minutes).

Arrange steak and vegetables on grill or broiler rack about 6 inches from heat source. Broil on medium heat until steak is cooked as desired, about 5 minutes each side for medium doneness.

Cook vegetables until they are tender, about 10 minutes, turning occasionally.

Thinly slice steak diagonally across the grain. Serve steak with vegetables and baked potato with sour cream.

Nutrition Facts

DINNER 3: STEAK WITH ZUCCHINI

PLAN	CALORIES	CARBS	PROTEIN	FAT	FIBER	SODIUM
1200	530	53	39	18	6	140
1500	630	62	49	21	7	170
1800	740	75	57	23	8	190

PORK CHOP WITH MUSHROOMS

Ingredients:

1–2½ tablespoons fresh green onion (1 to 2 stalks)

4 fresh mushrooms for 1200; 8 for 1500; 10 for 1800

¼ cup light, fat-free chicken stock for 1200; ⅓ cup for 1500; ½ cup for 1800

¼ teaspoon whole dried oregano

⅛ teaspoon table salt

⅛ teaspoon ground black pepper

7 ounces raw lean sirloin pork chop for 1200; 8 ounces for 1500; 9 ounces for 1800

7 ounces sweet potato with skin for 1200; 8 ounces for 1500; 10 ounces for 1800

1 cup chopped broccoli

Thinly slice green onions and chop mushrooms.

Heat the chicken stock in a medium skillet over medium heat.

Add green onions and cook for 1 minute; stir in mushrooms, oregano, salt and pepper. Cook and stir for an additional 2 minutes.

Place pork chop in skillet and brown both sides, about 7 minutes per side.

While pork chop is cooking, prepare sweet potato and broccoli. Pierce sweet potato several times with a fork and microwave on high 7–10 minutes until tender. Steam broccoli in microwave or on stovetop in water, until crisp-tender.

Serve pork chop with mushrooms, sweet potato and the side dish of broccoli.

Nutrition Facts

DINNER 4: PORK CHOP WITH MUSHROOMS

PLAN	CALORIES	CARBS	PROTEIN	FAT	FIBER	SODIUM
1200	490	49	50	8	9	620
1500	600	64	60	10	12	700
1800	680	72	67	11	13	810

TURKEY AND BEAN WRAPS

Ingredients:

Cooking spray

4 ounces 7% fat (93% lean) raw ground turkey breast for 1200; 5 ounces for 1500; 6 ounces for 1800

2 whole wheat tortillas (70 calories each)

¼ cup fat-free canned refried beans for 1200; ½ cup for 1500 and 1800

4 tablespoons shredded part skim mozzarella cheese for 1200 and 1500; ½ cup for 1800

½ cup shredded lettuce

½ chopped fresh tomato

2 tablespoons light sour cream

1 cup frozen or fresh green beans

Add cooking spray to skillet over medium heat and add ground turkey. Cook for 10 minutes or until turkey meat is browned.

Spread half of the refried beans and sprinkle half of the shredded cheese on each tortilla. Place tortillas on a microwave-safe plate and microwave for 15 seconds.

When ground turkey is done, drain the meat and divide it evenly between the 2 tortillas.

Add half the lettuce and tomato and 1 tablespoon of sour cream to each tortilla. Wrap up the tortillas and enjoy. Serve steamed green beans on the side.

Nutrition Facts

DINNER 5: TURKEY AND BEAN WRAPS

PLAN	CALORIES	CARBS	PROTEIN	FAT	FIBER	SODIUM
1200	510	42	50	19	19	1310
1500	580	50	59	21	22	1580
1800	710	51	71	29	21	1790

STEAK WITH RED PEPPER SAUCE

Ingredients:

6 ounces white potato for 1200; 7 ounces for 1500; 8 ounces for 1800

2–3 fresh garlic cloves

1 teaspoon olive oil

½ a medium-sized red bell pepper, sliced into ½" strips

½ chopped medium onion

½ cup fat-free beef broth

¼ teaspoon chopped fresh oregano

5½ ounces trimmed top loin strip steak for 1200; 7 ounces for 1500; 8 ounces for 1800

Pinch of salt

Black pepper to taste

5–7 asparagus spears

2 tablespoons light sour cream

Prepare potato by washing and piercing with a fork several times; microwave on high until tender, turning once halfway through cooking time (this may take 5–10 minutes).

In a large skillet, heat minced garlic in hot oil until fragrant. Add peppers and onion and cook for about 3 minutes. Add ¼ cup beef broth and oregano and cook until vegetables are crisp-tender and onions are translucent. Remove vegetables from skillet with a slotted spoon.

Season steak with salt and pepper and place into the skillet with remaining broth. Cook over medium-high heat about 4 minutes on each side or until desired doneness (145ºF for medium rare and 160ºF for medium). Transfer steak to a serving platter.

Add vegetables back to the skillet and heat through. Spoon vegetables and sauce over steak.

Trim ½" off the ends of the asparagus. Steam asparagus for 7 minutes or until done.

Serve steak with baked potato, topped with sour cream and the side dish of steamed asparagus.

Nutrition Facts

DINNER 6: STEAK WITH RED PEPPER SAUCE

PLAN	CALORIES	CARBS	PROTEIN	FAT	FIBER	SODIUM
1200	490	47	40	17	8	220
1500	600	58	50	20	10	250
1800	680	68	57	22	12	370

BEEF SESAME

Ingredients:

6½ ounces raw extra-lean beef tenderloin for 1200; 7½ ounces for 1500; 8½ ounces for 1800

1 teaspoon extra-virgin olive oil; 1½ teaspoons for 1800

1 tablespoon low-sodium soy sauce

½ tablespoon sesame seeds

1 tablespoon chopped green onion

Black pepper to taste

9 ounces sweet potato for 1200; 11 ounces for 1500; 13 ounces for 1800

1 cup frozen vegetables (blend of broccoli, carrots and water chestnuts) for 1200 and 1500; 1½ cups for 1800

1 teaspoon trans fat–free spread for 1200; 2 teaspoons for 1500 and 1800

Slice beef into thin strips, or purchase thinly sliced to save time.

Combine oil, soy sauce, sesame seeds, green onion and black pepper in a medium bowl and mix until well blended. Add in sliced beef and combine until beef is well coated. Cover and marinate in refrigerator 20 minutes or overnight if time allows.

Scrub sweet potato, pierce holes with a fork and bake in microwave until tender, approximately 7–10 minutes.

Heat vegetable blend as directed on package; sprinkle with favorite herbs if desired.

Heat skillet over medium-high heat until hot, but not smoking. Add beef and marinade to skillet and cook, occasionally stirring, until browned, about 3–4 minutes.

Cover sweet potato with trans fat–free spread.

Serve beef with sweet potato and vegetables.

Nutrition Facts

DINNER 7: BEEF SESAME

PLAN	CALORIES	CARBS	PROTEIN	FAT	FIBER	SODIUM
1200	490	46	41	15	9	650
1500	580	55	47	19	10	710
1800	680	66	54	23	12	770

CHICKEN STIR-FRY

Ingredients:

½ cup cooked brown rice for 1200; ¾ cup for 1500; 1 cup for 1800

⅓ cup canned mandarin oranges (in juice) for 1200 and 1500; ½ cup for 1800

1 tablespoon low-sodium soy sauce

6 ounces raw boneless, skinless chicken breast for 1200; 7 ounces for 1500; 8 ounces for 1800

2 teaspoons peanut oil (can use olive oil) for 1200; 1 tablespoon for 1500 and 1800

1 garlic clove

½ cup snow peas

¼ cup chopped green onion

½ cup sliced water chestnuts

Cook brown rice according to package directions.

Reserve 2 tablespoons of juice from mandarin oranges, drain the rest. Blend juice with soy sauce.

Slice chicken breast into strips. Heat 1 teaspoon of oil in frying pan over high heat. Add chicken and minced garlic to pan and stir-fry for 3 minutes or until chicken is done.

Add remaining oil and snow peas, green onion and water chestnuts and stir-fry for 3–5 minutes.

Add soy sauce mixture and cook, stirring to coat all ingredients with sauce. Stir in oranges just before serving. Serve chicken stir-fry over brown rice.

Nutrition Facts

DINNER 8: CHICKEN STIR-FRY

PLAN	CALORIES	CARBS	PROTEIN	FAT	FIBER	SODIUM
1200	490	46	45	13	6	510
1500	610	58	52	19	7	530
1800	720	73	60	20	8	550

DILL SALMON

Ingredients:

6 ounces red potato for 1200; 8 ounces for 1500; 10 ounces for 1800

3 tablespoons light sour cream

½ teaspoon fresh dill weed sprigs

⅛ teaspoon black pepper

1½ teaspoons Dijon mustard

1½ teaspoons white rice vinegar

½ teaspoon chopped green onion

5 ounces raw wild Atlantic salmon for 1200; 7 ounces for 1500; 8 ounces for 1800

½ teaspoon olive oil

1 cup green beans

Preheat grill or broiler on medium heat.

Prepare potato by washing and piercing with a fork several times. Microwave on high until tender, turning once halfway through cooking time for 5–10 minutes. Top with 1 tablespoon of sour cream when ready to serve.

Combine remaining 2 tablespoons of sour cream, dill, pepper, mustard, vinegar and green onion. Refrigerate until ready to serve.

Brush salmon with olive oil and grill (or broil) over hot coals for 5–8 minutes per side, depending on thickness, or until fish flakes easily with fork.

Steam green beans in microwave or on stovetop.

When salmon is done cooking, place it on a plate and top with dill sauce.

Serve dill salmon with baked potato and green beans.

Nutrition Facts

DINNER 9: DILL SALMON

PLAN	CALORIES	CARBS	PROTEIN	FAT	FIBER	SODIUM
1200	490	46	37	18	8	290
1500	620	58	49	21	9	320
1800	710	70	56	23	10	350

HAMBURGER OR CHEESEBURGER WITH CORN ON THE COB

Ingredients:

5 ounces raw 90% lean ground beef for 1200; 6 ounces for 1500; 6½ ounces for 1800

Pinch of salt and black pepper

Cooking spray

1 ounce slice low-fat cheese for 1500 and 1800 only

1 corn on the cob, 3" ear, or ½ cup frozen corn kernels for 1200 and 1500; 2 cobs or 1 cup for 1800

2 teaspoons trans fat–free spread for 1200 and 1500; 3 teaspoons for 1800

1 whole wheat hamburger bun

2 teaspoons ketchup

2 teaspoons mustard

Mix ground beef with pinch of salt and pepper; shape into patty about 1" thick. Either place on grill or pan fry with nonstick cooking spray over medium heat for 8 minutes on each side.

Add the slice of cheese at the end of cooking for the 1500- and 1800-calorie recipes.

While burger is cooking, husk the corn, pull off silky threads and cut out any blemishes with a pointed knife. Drop the corn into a large pot filled with boiling water. Cover the pot and let the water return to a boil again, then turn off the heat and keep the pot covered. After 5 minutes, remove the corn or keep warm in the water with heat off until ready to serve. If using frozen corn, heat in microwave.

Cover corn with trans fat–free spread.

Place cooked hamburger or cheeseburger in whole wheat hamburger bun. Brush with ketchup and mustard. Serve hamburger or cheeseburger with corn.

Nutrition Facts

DINNER 10: HAMBURGER OR CHEESEBURGER WITH CORN ON THE COB

PLAN	CALORIES	CARBS	PROTEIN	FAT	FIBER	SODIUM
1200	510	44	40	21	4	750
1500	600	45	48	27	4	870
1800	720	63	54	33	5	920

SPAGHETTI WITH MEAT SAUCE

Ingredients:

2 minced garlic cloves

1 teaspoon olive oil for 1200; 2 teaspoons for 1500 and 1800

6 ounces extra-lean ground sirloin beef for 1200; 7 ounces for 1500; 8 ounces for 1800

1 cup whole wheat pasta (cooked portion) for 1200; 1¼ cups for 1500; 1⅓ cups for 1800

½ cup jarred light tomato sauce for 1200; ⅔ cup for 1500; ¾ cup for 1800

1 cup cauliflower

Sauté garlic with oil in a skillet over medium heat. Add ground sirloin and cook until meat is well browned.

While meat is cooking, place water in a pot to boil for pasta. Once water is boiling add pasta and cook until done.

Heat the tomato sauce over medium heat until warm.

Add tomato sauce to meat mixture and serve over cooked spaghetti. Serve with steamed cauliflower on the side.

Nutrition Facts

DINNER 11: SPAGHETTI WITH MEAT SAUCE

PLAN	CALORIES	CARBS	PROTEIN	FAT	FIBER	SODIUM
1200	500	54	45	13	11	500
1500	610	63	52	19	12	650
1800	690	68	56	25	24	1420

TURKEY CHILI

Ingredients:

Cooking spray

4 ounces of 7% fat ground turkey for 1200; 5 ounces of 4% fat for 1500; 6 ounces of 4% fat for 1800

¼ chopped large white onion

2 cloves chopped fresh garlic

2½ teaspoons olive oil

½ cup drained and rinsed canned kidney beans (any type) for 1200;
¾ cup for 1500; 1 cup for 1800

¾ cup canned crushed tomatoes for 1200; 1 cup for 1500 and 1800

½ teaspoon dried basil

1 teaspoon chili powder

¼ chopped large green bell pepper

⅓ to ½ pound (4–6 cups) fresh spinach

Add nonstick cooking spray to pan and cook ground turkey over medium heat for 10 minutes or until turkey is browned. Drain meat and set aside, keep warm.

Cook onion and half of the chopped garlic in oil in a medium saucepan over low heat for 6 minutes. Add ground turkey, kidney beans, tomatoes, basil, chili powder and green pepper. Cover, adjust heat to a simmer and cook 10 minutes.

Sauté spinach and remaining garlic in a skillet with nonstick cooking spray over medium-high heat until spinach wilts.

Serve turkey chili with spinach on the side.

Nutrition Facts

DINNER 12: TURKEY CHILI

PLAN	CALORIES	CARBS	PROTEIN	FAT	FIBER	SODIUM
1200	500	53	36	20	19	940
1500	610	67	46	22	25	1230
1800	700	76	55	24	28	1430

SHRIMP SAUTÉ

Ingredients:

¾ cup cooked brown rice for 1200; 1 cup for 1500; 1¼ cups for 1800

6 ounces raw (or thawed frozen) uncooked shelled shrimp for 1200; 7 ounces for 1500; 8 ounces for 1800

1 teaspoon finely chopped fresh parsley

1 teaspoon finely chopped fresh rosemary

1 minced garlic clove

¼ teaspoon fresh thyme

1 teaspoon olive oil for 1200 and 1500; 1½ teaspoons for 1800

1 teaspoon lemon juice

2 fluid ounces low-sodium chicken stock

1 teaspoon trans fat–free spread

⅛ teaspoon black pepper

1 cup fresh broccoli

Cook brown rice according to package directions.

In a medium bowl, toss the shrimp with the parsley, rosemary, garlic, thyme and half of the olive oil. Set aside for 15 minutes.

Place the remaining oil in a medium nonstick skillet and heat over medium-high heat. Add the shrimp along with the marinade. Sauté, stirring constantly, until shrimp are cooked through, about 3–5 minutes. Place shrimp over bed of hot cooked brown rice and keep warm.

Add the lemon juice and 1 ounce (approximately 2 tablespoons) of chicken stock to the skillet, scraping up any browned bits from the bottom. Cook over medium-high heat, stirring frequently, until reduced by half. Add the trans fat–free spread and continue to cook until melted.

Pour sauce over shrimp and brown rice, season with pepper and serve hot.

Steam broccoli in microwave or on stovetop in remaining 1 ounce (approximately 2 tablespoons) of chicken stock.

Serve shrimp sauté with steamed broccoli.

Nutrition Facts
DINNER 13: SHRIMP SAUTÉ

PLAN	CALORIES	CARBS	PROTEIN	FAT	FIBER	SODIUM
1200	500	50	44	13	8	440
1500	580	62	51	14	9	480
1800	690	73	58	18	10	530

PORK CHOP AND BUTTERNUT SQUASH

Ingredients:

¼ teaspoon crushed dried rosemary

¼ teaspoon dried basil

¼ teaspoon minced garlic

Pinch of black pepper

2 teaspoons olive oil for 1200 and 1800; 1 tablespoon for 1500

6 ounces raw lean sirloin pork chop for 1200; 7 ounces for 1500; 8 ounces for 1800

¼ cup lemon juice

8 ounces frozen butternut squash for 1200; 12 ounces for 1500; 14 ounces for 1800

Ground cinnamon to taste

8–10 asparagus spears

In a small bowl, stir together rosemary, basil, garlic and pepper.

Heat olive oil in a large skillet over medium heat.

Dip pork chop in lemon juice and sprinkle both sides with herb mixture. Place pork chop in skillet and brown both sides, about 7 minutes per side.

Microwave package of frozen butternut squash for 9 minutes or until done. Once cooked, sprinkle squash with cinnamon to taste.

Trim ½" off the ends of the asparagus. Steam asparagus for 7 minutes or until done.

Serve pork chop with steamed asparagus and cooked butternut squash.

Nutrition Facts

DINNER 14: PORK CHOP AND BUTTERNUT SQUASH

PLAN	CALORIES	CARBS	PROTEIN	FAT	FIBER	SODIUM
1200	500	41	46	15	5	170
1500	602	53	53	15	6	160
1800	690	69	62	22	6	240

CAJUN TILAPIA

Ingredients:

¾ cup cooked brown rice for 1200; 1 cup for 1500; 1⅓ cups for 1800

7 ounces raw tilapia for 1200; 8 ounces for 1500; 9 ounces for 1800

Salt-free Cajun spice blend to taste

Cooking spray

1 tablespoon extra-virgin olive oil

2 minced garlic cloves

⅓ pound (4 cups) fresh spinach

Cook brown rice according to package directions.

While rice is cooking, sprinkle tilapia with Cajun spice blend to taste. Spray sauté pan with cooking spray and cook tilapia over medium heat for 3 minutes on each side.

In another pan, add olive oil and minced garlic and cook until fragrant (about 30 seconds). Add spinach and cook until wilted.

Serve tilapia over the brown rice with sautéed spinach on the side.

Nutrition Facts

DINNER 15: CAJUN TILAPIA

PLAN	CALORIES	CARBS	PROTEIN	FAT	FIBER	SODIUM
1200	510	40	45	19	3	130
1500	610	53	52	20	3	160
1800	720	70	60	21	4	170

OMELET LAVASH WRAP

Ingredients:

¼ chopped red bell pepper for 1200; ½ for 1500 and 1800

¼ chopped medium onion

¼ cup sliced mushrooms

2 teaspoons canola oil

2 large eggs for 1200 and 1500; 3 eggs for 1800

2 tablespoons nonfat milk for 1200 and 1500; ¼ cup skim milk for 1800

Cooking spray

¼ cup shredded mozzarella cheese for 1200; ½ cup for 1500 and 1800

1 Joseph's whole grain lavash bread

1 cup diced melon for 1200; 1¼ cups for 1500; 1½ cups for 1800

Sauté red pepper, onion and mushrooms in oil over medium-high heat for 2–3 minutes. Remove vegetables from the pan and set aside.

Combine eggs and milk in a small bowl and whisk. Add cooking spray to pan. On medium heat, scramble eggs until cooked through. Add cooked vegetables to the pan and combine with scrambled eggs.

Sprinkle cheese on lavash bread and add egg and vegetable mixture on top. Wrap and serve with side of melon.

Nutrition Facts

DINNER 16: OMELET LAVASH WRAP

PLAN	CALORIES	CARBS	PROTEIN	FAT	FIBER	SODIUM
1200	500	41	36	29	13	980
1500	600	46	44	34	13	1070
1800	690	50	50	40	13	1290

VEGETABLE-ONLY OR TURKEY-AND-VEGETABLE LASAGNA

Ingredients:

Cooking spray

⅛ cup chopped onion for 1200 and 1500; ¼ cup for 1800

1 chopped garlic clove

½ cup sliced mushrooms

Ground black pepper to taste

1 tablespoon salt-free Italian seasoning

¼ cup ricotta cheese

1 egg

½ cup heated and drained frozen chopped spinach

1 cup crushed/diced tomatoes for 1200; 1¼ cups for 1500; 1½ cups for 1800

1 ounce no-boil lasagna noodles for 1200; 1½ ounces for 1500; 2 ounces for 1800

¼ cup part-skim mozzarella cheese for 1200 and 1500; ⅓ cup for 1800

2 ounces of 7% fat ground turkey for 1500 and 1800 only (leave out of vegetable lasagna for 1200)

Vegetable Only: Preheat oven to 375°F. Spray a skillet with cooking spray.

Over medium heat, cook onion and garlic until soft. Add mushrooms, black pepper and Italian seasoning to taste.

While onions and mushrooms are cooking, mix ricotta cheese and egg together in a small bowl. Mix spinach into ricotta cheese mixture.

Season tomatoes with Italian seasoning as desired.

In a square casserole dish or baking pan spread ⅓ of the tomatoes along the bottom. Layer lasagna noodles, then ricotta cheese mixture, then mushroom mixture, and then tomatoes evenly between layers. Cover top of lasagna with mozzarella cheese.

Cover with aluminum foil, place in oven and bake for approximately 45 minutes until lasagna is bubbling and cheese is brown.

Turkey and Vegetable: Preheat oven to 375°F. Spray a skillet with cooking spray.

Over medium heat, cook onion and garlic until soft. Add ground turkey, seasoning with black pepper and Italian seasoning to taste. When ground turkey is almost cooked through, add mushrooms to skillet.

While turkey and mushroom mixture are cooking, mix ricotta cheese and egg together in a small bowl. Mix spinach into ricotta cheese mixture.

Season tomatoes with Italian seasoning as desired.

In a square casserole dish or baking pan, spread ¼ of the tomatoes along the bottom. Layer lasagna noodles, then ricotta cheese mixture, then mushroom and ground turkey mixture, and then tomatoes evenly between layers. Cover top of lasagna with mozzarella cheese.

Cover with aluminum foil, place in oven and bake for approximately 45 minutes until lasagna is bubbling and cheese is brown.

Nutrition Facts

DINNER 17: VEGETABLE-ONLY OR TURKEY-AND-VEGETABLE LASAGNA

PLAN	CALORIES	CARBS	PROTEIN	FAT	FIBER	SODIUM
1200	480	49	34	18	9	800
1500	630	66	49	22	11	940
1800	730	80	54	24	13	1110

ACCEPTABLE FROZEN DINNERS (LISTED BY BRAND AND PRODUCT LINE)

We aim to have you eat 2 frozen meals for dinner. In an effort to do this, the nutrient targets are as follows for each meal:

Total Calories: 250–300
Total Carbohydrates: <35 g
Total Protein: >15 g
   (the higher you can find the better)
Total Fat: <7 g
Total Sodium: <650 mg

Sometimes people want to mix and match a higher calorie meal with a lower calorie one. If this is the case, aim for these targets for the whole dinner:

Total Calories: 600
Total Carbohydrates: 60–70 g
Total Protein: 30–45 g
   (try to find choices that are at least 20 g of protein)
Total Fat: <15 g
Total Sodium: <1200 mg

The following are some examples of good frozen dinner choices listed by brand and product line. Bear in mind that the selections change frequently, so if you have trouble finding these, just refer to the guidelines above as you decide which meals to buy.

HEALTHY CHOICE TOP CHEF CAFÉ STEAMERS

PRODUCT	CALORIES	CARBOHYDRATE			PROTEIN		FAT		SODIUM
		g	% Cal	Fiber	g	% Cal	g	% Cal	mg
Chicken Linguini with Red Pepper Alfredo	260	28	43	5	22	34	6	21	510
Grilled Chicken Pesto with Vegetables	310	34	44	3	21	27	9	26	550
Chicken Fresca with Chardonnay	240	30	50	4	16	27	6	23	570
Roasted Chicken Marsala with Mushrooms	240	29	48	4	18	30	5	19	420

HEALTHY CHOICE MEDITERRANEAN INSPIRED CAFÉ STEAMERS

PRODUCT	CALORIES	CARBOHYDRATE			PROTEIN		FAT		SODIUM
		g	% Cal	Fiber	g	% Cal	g	% Cal	mg
Grilled Basil Chicken	270	35	52	6	18	27	6	20	500

HEALTHY CHOICE SELECT ENTRÉES

PRODUCT	CALORIES	CARBOHYDRATE			PROTEIN		FAT		SODIUM
		g	% Cal	Fiber	g	% Cal	g	% Cal	mg
Bacon & Smokey Cheddar Chicken	250	31	50	2	17	27	6	22	520
Chicken Alfredo Florentine	220	28	51	4	16	31	4.5	18	560

HEALTHY CHOICE COMPLETE MEALS

PRODUCT	CALORIES	CARBOHYDRATE			PROTEIN		FAT		SODIUM
		g	% Cal	Fiber	g	% Cal	g	% Cal	mg
Sundried Tomato and Chicken Alfredo	270	31	46	5	23	34	7	23	430
Beef Strips Portabello	280	35	50	7	18	26	7	23	560
Beef Bourbon Dijon	280	33	47	6	20	29	7	23	600
Beef Pot Roast	250	32	51	5	17	27	6	22	500
Chicken Pesto Alfredo	310	36	46	7	24	31	7	20	500

KASHI

PRODUCT	CALORIES	CARBOHYDRATE			PROTEIN		FAT		SODIUM
		g	% Cal	Fiber	g	% Cal	g	% Cal	mg
Chicken Florentine	270	31	45	5	22	32	9	30	550

SMART ONES

PRODUCT	CALORIES	CARBOHYDRATE			PROTEIN		FAT		SODIUM
		g	% Cal	Fiber	g	% Cal	g	% Cal	mg
Chicken Marsala	250	30	48	5	24	38	3.5	13	640

LEAN CUISINE MARKET COLLECTION

PRODUCT	CALORIES	CARBOHYDRATE			PROTEIN		FAT		SODIUM
		g	% Cal	Fiber	g	% Cal	g	% Cal	mg
Steak Tips Dijon	280	35	50	5	18	26	7	23	600

LEAN CUISINE SPA CUISINE

PRODUCT	CALORIES	CARBOHYDRATE			PROTEIN		FAT		SODIUM
		g	% Cal	Fiber	g	% Cal	g	% Cal	mg
Hunan Stir Fry with Beef	280	36	51	5	16	23	8	26	460
Lemongrass Chicken	260	33	51	5	19	29	6	21	550
Rosemary Chicken	210	27	51	5	16	30	4	17	510
Salmon with Basil	210	25	48	5	15	29	6	26	590

LEAN CUISINE CULINARY COLLECTION

PRODUCT	CALORIES	CARBOHYDRATE			PROTEIN		FAT		SODIUM
		g	% Cal	Fiber	g	% Cal	g	% Cal	mg
Chicken Carbonara	270	33	49	3	21	31	6	20	600
Chicken in Peanut Sauce	280	35	50	5	21	30	6	19	550
Chicken Marsala	220	25	45	2	17	31	6	25	620
Chicken with Basil Cream Sauce	230	28	49	2	16	29	6	23	510

continued

Chicken with Lasagna Rollatini	290	34	47	3	18	25	9	28	560
Fiesta Grilled Chicken	260	33	51	4	19	29	6	20	600
Glazed Chicken	240	26	43	2	22	37	5	19	450
Grilled Chicken Caesar	240	30	50	3	17	32	6	23	530
Meatloaf with Mashed Potatoes	250	25	40	3	20	32	8	29	590
Salisbury Steak with Macaroni & Cheese	260	23	35	3	23	35	8	28	540
Sun Dried Tomato Pesto Chicken	270	28	41	4	18	27	9	30	570

The daily calories in your Diabetes Breakthrough meal plan are based on research compiled by the Joslin Diabetes Center and others about the most beneficial distribution of carbohydrate, protein and fat (macronutrients) in your diet for management of body weight and prevention and management of type 2 diabetes. These nutritional guidelines are recommended if: you are overweight or obese; have a weight circumference of 35 inches (88 cm) or higher for women or 40 inches (102 cm) or more for men; have type 2 diabetes or prediabetes; or are at high risk for type 2 diabetes or metabolic syndrome. These guidelines are included for your reference.

General Guidelines:
- There is strong evidence that weight reduction improves insulin sensitivity, glycemic control, lipid profile and blood pressure in type 2 diabetes and decreases the risk of developing type 2 diabetes in prediabetes and high-risk populations.
- To select an approach for medical nutrition therapy, target individuals should be referred to a registered dietitian (RD) or a qualified health care provider for assessment and review of medical management and treatment goals.
- Priorities of medical nutrition therapy for this population include:
  - Weight reduction
  - Meal-to-meal consistency in carbohydrate distribution for those with fixed medication/insulin programs
  - Consideration of other nutrition-related comorbidities such as hypertension and dyslipidemia
- The meal plan composition, described below, is for general guidance only and may be individualized by the RD or other health care provider according to clinical judgment, individual (patient) preferences and needs and metabolic response. The plan should

be reevaluated and modified to respond to changes in parameters such as blood pressure, A1C and frequency of hypo/hyperglycemia. Modification of goals may be needed for those requiring additional dietary considerations such as those with hyperkalemia or those who are vegetarian.

Weight Reduction:

- A structured lifestyle plan that combines dietary modification and exercise is necessary for weight reduction.
- A modest and gradual weight reduction of 1 pound every one to two weeks should be the optimal target.
- Reduction of daily calories should range between 250 to 500 calories. Total daily caloric intake should not be less than 1000–1200 for women and 1200–1600 for men, or based on an RD assessment of usual intake.
- A 5–10 percent weight loss may result in significant improvement in blood glucose control among patients with diabetes and help prevent the onset of diabetes among individuals with prediabetes. Weight reduction should be individualized and continued until an agreed upon BMI and/or other metabolic goals are reached.
- Target individuals should meet with an RD to learn and practice portion control as an effective way of weight control.
- Meal replacements (MR) in the form of shakes, bars, ready-to-eat powders and prepackaged meals that match these nutrition guidelines may be effective in initiating and maintaining weight loss.
  - Meal replacements should be used under the supervision of an RD.
  - When meal replacements are initiated, glucose levels should be carefully monitored and, if needed, antihyperglycemic medications should be adjusted.
  - Meal replacements should be used with caution by those with hyperkalemia.
- Bariatric surgeries, although not without medical and nutrition risks, are effective options and may be discussed when indicated (consider

in individuals with BMI >40 kg/m² and those with BMI >35 kg/m² with other comorbidities). To date, there is limited evidence to support the recommendation of bariatric surgeries for patients with BMI <35 kg/m² even if they have diabetes or other comorbid conditions.

MACRONUTRIENT COMPOSITION

Fat	Percentage	There is general agreement that fat quality rather than quantity is important. The total fat intake should be generally limited to less than 35 percent of total daily caloric intake. Saturated fat should be limited to <7 percent of total caloric intake. Polyunsaturated and monounsaturated fats should comprise the rest of the fat intake. Cholesterol limited to <300 mg/day or <200 mg/day in individuals with LDL-cholesterol >100 mg/dl.
	Recommended	Mono and polyunsaturated fats (e.g., olive oil, canola oil, nuts/seeds, avocado and fish, particularly those high in omega-3 fatty acids); 4 ounces of oily fish (e.g., salmon, herring, trout, sardines, fresh tuna) 2 times/week, as a source of omega-3 fatty acids.
	Not Recommended	Foods high in saturated fat, including beef, pork, lamb and high-fat dairy products (e.g., cream cheese, whole milk or yogurt); foods high in trans fats (e.g., fast foods, commercially baked goods, some margarines); foods high in dietary cholesterol, such as egg yolks and organ meats.
	Cholesterol	<300 mg/day or <200 mg/day for individuals with LDL-cholesterol >100 mg/dl. Egg yolks should be limited to 2 or 3 per week; other foods high in dietary cholesterol, such as red meat, whole-fat dairy products, shellfish and organ meats should be limited, as well.
Protein	Percentage	Protein intake should not be less than 1.2 g/kg of adjusted body weight. Adjusted Body Weight = IBW (Ideal Body Weight) + 0.25 (Current Weight = IBW). This amount generally accounts for 20–30 percent of total caloric intake. There are no reliable scientific findings to support a protein intake that exceeds 2 g/kg of adjusted body weight.

continued

MACRONUTRIENT COMPOSITION

Protein (continued)	Percentage (continued)	Emerging data suggests that protein aids in the sensation of fullness (low-protein meal plans are associated with increased hunger). A modest increase in protein reduces appetite and assists in achieving and maintaining weight reduction. Protein also helps to minimize loss of lean body mass.
	Recommended	Fish, skinless poultry, nonfat or low-fat dairy, nuts, seeds and legumes.
	Not Recommended	High-saturated-fat protein sources in excess (e.g., beef, pork, lamb and high-fat dairy products), as they may be associated with increased cardiovascular risk.
	Patients with Renal Issues	Although reducing total calories may result in a reduction of the absolute total amount of protein intake, patients with signs of kidney disease (i.e., one or more of the following: proteinuria, GFR<60 ml/min) should consult a nephrologist before increasing total or percentage protein in their diet. Protein intake for these patients should be modified, but not lowered to a level that may jeopardize their overall health or increase their risk of malnutrition or hypoalbuminemia.
Carbohydrate	Percentage	Intake should be adjusted to meet the cultural and food preferences of the individual.
		The total daily intake of carbohydrate should be at least 130 g/day and ideally 40–45 percent of the total caloric intake.
	Consideration of Glycemic Index/ Glycemic Load	The glycemic index/glycemic load is an important factor that patients should apply in their daily selection of carbohydrate foods. Foods with a low glycemic index should be selected (e.g., whole grains, legumes, fruits, green salad with olive oil-based dressing and most vegetables).
	Recommended	Vegetables and fruits, legumes, whole and minimally processed grains.
	Not Recommended	Sugar, refined carbohydrates, processed grains and starchy foods, especially sugary beverages, most pastas, white bread, white rice, low-fiber cereal and white potatoes, should be consumed in limited quantities.

| Fiber | Approximately 14 g of fiber/1000 calories (20–35 g) per day is recommended. If tolerated, approximately 50 g/day is effective in improving postprandial hyperglycemia and should be encouraged. |
| | Fiber from unprocessed food, such as vegetables, fruits, seeds, nuts and legumes is preferable but, if needed, fiber supplements such as psyllium, resistant starch and β-glucan. |

MICRONUTRIENT COMPOSITION

Sodium	Daily consumption should be <2300 mg (about 1 teaspoon of salt) per day. Further reduction to 1500 mg is recommended in people >50 years of age including those with chronic kidney disease.
	Slow acclimatization to lower sodium intake is advisable.
Potassium	Daily consumption should be a minimum of 4,700 mg unless potassium excretion is impaired.
	Potassium helps offset high sodium intake by triggering more sodium excretion by the kidneys.
	Potassium-rich foods include fruits and vegetables like bananas, mushrooms, spinach and almonds.

Dietary Supplements:
- In individuals who are not deficient, data do not support the use of vitamins or minerals to improve glucose control or the use of herbal supplements or spices to improve glucose control.

Non-Nutritive Sweeteners:
- All FDA-approved non-nutritive sweeteners are permissible in moderate quantities (e.g., one diet soda daily).

Alcohol:
- If consumed, alcohol intake must be moderate. No more than 1 drink a day for women and no more than 2 drinks a day for men

(one drink is equal to 12 ounces of regular beer, 5 ounces of wine or 1½ ounces of 80-proof distilled alcohol).

- Alcoholic beverages contain calories and are low in nutritional value.
- It is not advisable to increase alcohol consumption for the purpose of deriving purported health benefit.

Exercise and Behavioral Modification:
- Exercise should be included in the nutrition prescription described above. Exercise should be an integral component of any weight reduction plan as it helps maximize the benefits of weight reduction on diabetes control and may prevent coronary and cerebral vascular disease.
- 60–90 minutes of moderately intensive activity, at least five days of the week, is encouraged for weight loss, unless contraindicated.
- Exercise program should include a mix of aerobic and resistance training to maintain or increase lean body mass, as well as stretching.

Suggested Macronutrient Distribution According to Clinical Guideline

CALORIE LEVEL	CARBOHYDRATE		PROTEIN		FAT	
	Grams	%	Grams	%	Grams	%
1000	130	~50*	75	30	27	20
1200	135	45	75–90	25–30	40	30
1500	150–170	40–45	75–110	20–30	50	30
1800	180–200	40–45	90–135	20–30	60	30
2000	200–225	40–45	100–150	20–30	70	~30

*A minimum of 130 grams of carbohydrate per day, in a 1000-calorie meal plan, calculates to approximately 50 percent of the total daily calories.

Adapted from Joslin Diabetes Center education materials.

It is important that you consult with your health care provider in order to effectively make changes to your medication types and/or doses during this program. Do not attempt to make any of these adjustments on your own. We have included the Joslin Diabetes Center Why WAIT program medication algorithms for you to provide to them. These are for the sole use of your health care provider while they are assisting you with making these critical decisions.

Diabetes Medications and Body Weight				
1. IDENTIFY	**Weight Gain ↑**		**Weight Neutral →**	**Weight Loss ↓**
	Significant	Modest		
2. PLAN	Pioglitazone (Actos) Rosiglitazone (Avandia) Sulfonylureas Glyburide Glipizide Insulin NPH Glargine (Lantus, Toujeo) Regular Aspart (Novolog) Lispro (Humalog) Glulisine (Apidra) Afrezza (inhaled insulin)	Sulfonylurea Glimepiride Glipizide XL Glinides Repaglinide (Prandin) Nateglinide (Starlix) Insulin Demetir (Levemir) Short-acting (Postprandial)	Metformin DPP-4 Inhibitors Sitagliptin (Januvia) Saxagliptin (Onglyza) Linagliptin (Tradjenta) Alogliptin (Nesina) α-Glucosidase Inhibitors Acarbose (Precose) Miglitol (Glycet) Colesevelam (Welchol) Bromocriptine (Cycloset)	GLP-1 Analogs Exenatide (Byetta) Exenatide ER (Bydureon) Liraglutide (Victoza) Dulaglutide (Trulicity) Albiglutide (Tanzeum/ Eperzan) Lixisenatide (Lyxumia) Pramlintide (Symlin) Canagliflozin (Invokana) Dapagliflozin (Farxiga, Forxiga) Empagliflozin (Jardiance)
3. CHANGE	Stop, Reduce or Switch		Continue	Add

During the 12-week Diabetes Breakthrough program itself, your health care provider is advised to follow these medication recommendations in making adjustments to your medications to optimize your weight loss and blood glucose control:

Algorithm for Medical Management for Type 2 Diabetes Mellitus

Why WAIT Program: First 12 Weeks

Goal is to use metformin and GLP-1 analog/DPP-4 inhibitors at highest doses possible and use SFU/TZD/insulin sparingly, in that order of preferred usage. For those on insulin, concomitant pramlinitide is preferred; short-acting insulin will be dosed postprandially.

Medication changes can be made weekly based on BG logs

On Oral Diabetes Medications		On Insulin	
HbA1c < 8% or eAG < 180 mg/dl	**HbA1c > 8%** or eAG ≥ 180 mg/dl	**HbA1c < 8%** or eAG < 180 mg/dl	**HbA1c = 8%** or eAG = 180 mg/dl
Metformin: add, continue at same dose or increase to max dose (2500 mg QD) as tolerated	Metformin: add, continue or increase to max dose (2500 mg QD) as tolerated	If on ≤ 20 units daily dose, stop insulin, add GLP-1 analog	Change long-acting insulin to detemir, adjust dose
Sulfonylurea: stop or reduce dose	May add GLP-1 agonist	If on > 20 units daily dose: change long-acting basal insulin to detemir, reduce insulin dose by 20 units & add GLP-1 analog	Add GLP-1 analog
TZD: stop or reduce dose	Sulfonylurea: may add or change to long-acting forms (glimepiride, glipizide XL)	Add short-acting insulin and stop GLP-1 analog	Add short-acting insulin and stop GLP-1 analog
May add GLP-1 analog	TZD: stop or reduce dose	May add pramlintide; titrate to 120 mcg TID	Add pramlintide
If GLP-1 analog not covered by insurance, may add DPP-4 inhibitor	If GLP-1 analog not covered by insurance, may add DPP-4 inhibitor	Titrate insulin based on FBG and PPBG	
If hypoglycemia develops	**HbA1c = 8%** or eAG = 180 mg/dl	Metformin may be added to insulin	
Reduce or stop SFU	Continue GLP-1 (or DPP-4 inhibitor). Maximize SFU and/or add detemir insulin	If HbA1c < 6.5% or eAG < 140 mg/dl, reduce/stop short-acting insulin ± reduce/stop long-acting insulin. May add back OHA. If insulin stopped, pramlintide will be stopped, and may add back GLP-1 analog.	
Decrease metformin dose			
Decrease GLP-1 analog/ DPP-4 inhibitor dose			

After you have finished the 12-week Diabetes Breakthrough program, your health care team is advised to follow these recommended changes:

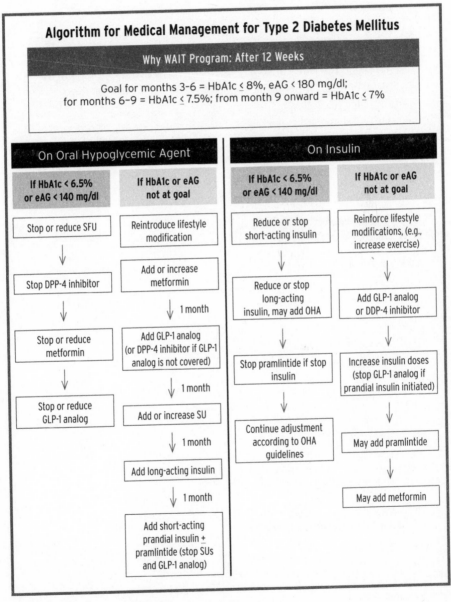

Algorithm for Medical Management for Type 2 Diabetes Mellitus

Why WAIT Program: After 12 Weeks

Goal for months 3–6 = HbA1c ≤ 8%, eAG < 180 mg/dl;
for months 6–9 = HbA1c ≤ 7.5%; from month 9 onward = HbA1c ≤ 7%

On Oral Hypoglycemic Agent		On Insulin	
If HbA1c < 6.5% or eAG < 140 mg/dl	**If HbA1c or eAG not at goal**	**If HbA1c < 6.5% or eAG < 140 mg/dl**	**If HbA1c or eAG not at goal**
Stop or reduce SFU	Reintroduce lifestyle modification	Reduce or stop short-acting insulin	Reinforce lifestyle modifications, (e.g., increase exercise)
↓	↓	↓	↓
Stop DPP-4 inhibitor	Add or increase metformin	Reduce or stop long-acting insulin, may add OHA	Add GLP-1 analog or DDP-4 inhibitor
↓	↓ 1 month	↓	↓
Stop or reduce metformin	Add GLP-1 analog (or DPP-4 inhibitor if GLP-1 analog is not covered)	Stop pramlintide if stop insulin	Increase insulin doses (stop GLP-1 analog if prandial insulin initiated)
↓	↓ 1 month	↓	↓
Stop or reduce GLP-1 analog	Add or increase SU	Continue adjustment according to OHA guidelines	May add pramlintide
	↓ 1 month		↓
	Add long-acting insulin		May add metformin
	↓ 1 month		
	Add short-acting prandial insulin + pramlintide (stop SUs and GLP-1 analog)		

Turkey and Bean Wraps, 285

Turkey Chili, 291–92

Vegetable-Only or Turkey-and-Vegetable Lasagna, 296–98

Disqualifying the positive, 186

Doctors. *See* Health care team

DPP-4 inhibitors, 75, *76,* 79, *82,* 83, 128, *310*

Drinks, 44

Drugs. *See* Diabetes medications; Insulin

Dulaglutide (Trulicity), *72,* 75, *76,* 83, 131–32, *309*

Dumbbells Press, 143

E

Eating out. *See* Restaurants

Eating patterns, 65, 147–52, 192, 213

Elevated blood glucose. *See* Hyperglycemia

Emotional eating, 65, 213, 216, 225

mindful eating vs., 226–28

Empagliflozin (Jardiance), *72,* 73, 75, *76, 82,* 129, *309*

Eperzan (albiglutide), 72, 75, *76,* 131–32, *309*

Equipment and supplies, 25–26, 141

European restaurants, *208*

Exercise

amount of, 258–59

barriers to, 60–64, 199–200, 244

best time for, 53

blood glucose and, 7–8, 48, 98–100, 116–17, 156, 162

checkup before, 18

counting daily steps, 259–62

dropout rate, 198

health benefits of, 7–8, 18–19, 49, 172

injuries, preventing and treating, 103–5

intensity of, 52–53

logbook for, 54–55, 60

physical activity vs., 47–48

plans. *See* Exercise plans

safety precautions, 60, 100–102

scheduling, 200–201

types of, 49–50. *See also specific types of exercise*

warm up and cool down, 50–51

weight control registry and, 234–36, 235

weight maintenance training options, 257–58

when to or not to, 53, 100, 103

Exercise clothes, 25, 30–31, 60

Exercise equipment, 25–26, 141

Exercise plans, xv, 10, 18–21, 51, 105–6

safety checklist, 60

Week 1, *19,* 52, *52,* 54

Week 2, 96, *96–97, 191*

Week 3, 121, *121*

Week 4, *20,* 140, *141*

Week 5, 20, 163–64, *164*

Week 6, *20,* 173, *173*

Week 7, *20,* 196, *196–97*

Week 8, *20,* 205, *205*

Week 9, *20,* 219, *220*

Week 10, *21,* 229, *229*

Week 11, *21,* 237, *238*

Week 12, *21,* 245, *245*

Week 13 and beyond, 256, *256–57*

Extensors Stretch, 58

Eyes, xiii, 14, 18, 101, 160, 161

F

Fad diets. *See* Diets, fad

Falls (falling), 204–5

Family and friends, influence of, 191–96, 201–2, 251–52, 255

ABOUT THE AUTHORS

Osama Hamdy, M.D., Ph.D., is one of the faces of the Joslin Diabetes Center, the world's preeminent diabetes research and clinical care organization affiliated with Harvard Medical School. He is the founder and medical director of the Joslin obesity clinical program, director of inpatient diabetes management and assistant professor of medicine at Harvard Medical School. He is the creator of Joslin Why WAIT program, the world's first clinical program designed to help patients with diabetes lose weight through a novel multidisciplinary approach. An international diabetes and weight loss expert, he completed his medical and doctoral training at Mansoura University in Mansoura, Egypt, followed by fellowships at the University of Missouri Hospital and Clinics and Harvard University Joslin Diabetes Center. He chaired the task force that developed Joslin's nutrition guidelines, is a member of the Nutrition Committee of the American Association of Clinical Endocrinologists and vice-chair of International Transcultural Diabetes Nutrition Working Group and has published more than 150 research articles and book chapters accessible at www.ohamdy.com.

Sheri R. Colberg, Ph.D., is a professor of exercise science at Old Dominion University and an adjunct professor of internal medicine at Eastern Virginia Medical School. With expertise in exercise, diabetes, aging and weight loss, she has worked with hundreds of individuals prescribing a variety of physical activity, diabetes management and weight loss techniques. A funded diabetes researcher, she is also the author of more than 250 research and educational articles, 13 book chapters and nine books, including *Diabetic Athlete's Handbook, The 7 Step Diabetes Fitness Plan, 50 Secrets of the Longest Living People with Diabetes, The Science of Staying Young* and *Exercise and Diabetes:*

A Clinician's Guide to Prescribing Physical Activity. A graduate of Stanford University and the University of California, Davis and Berkeley, she is widely considered an international expert in exercise, diabetes and disease prevention through lifestyle and behavioral changes. She has also been living exceptionally well with diabetes for over four and a half decades. Visit her website at www.SheriColberg.com.

CONTRIBUTING AUTHORS

Jacqueline I. Shahar, MEd, RCEP, CDE, is a clinical exercise physiologist, certified diabetes educator and the manager of the exercise physiology department at the Joslin Diabetes Center. She designed the innovative exercise program used in the Joslin Why WAIT program and serves as its lead exercise physiologist. She served in the Israeli Defense Force as a fitness combat trainer and then graduated from the Kibbutzim College of Education in Tel Aviv, Israel. After earning her master's degree in applied exercise science from Springfield College, she completed her internship at the Joslin Diabetes Center. She consults on exercise and diabetes, teaches group classes and trains health care providers.

Ann Goebel-Fabbri, Ph.D., is an assistant professor of psychiatry at Harvard Medical School. Her role at the Joslin Diabetes Center integrates teaching, research and treatment focused on disordered eating behaviors in patients with type 1 and type 2 diabetes, which include food and insulin restriction, binge eating and obesity. She designed the behavioral intervention for the Joslin Why WAIT and the Joslin YOU-Turn programs, remains the leading psychologist for the Why WAIT program and provides individualized treatment for participants in both programs.

Gillian Arathuzik, RD, LDN, CDE, is a nutrition diabetes educator at the Joslin Diabetes Center. She designed the menus and meal plans for the Joslin

Why WAIT program and serves as the lead dietitian for the program. Recently, she was a coauthor of the book *Prevention's Flat Belly Diet for Diabetes.* Having received her BS in nutrition and dietetics at the University of Vermont and completed her dietetic internship at Indiana University Medical Center, she is also certified in adult weight management through the American Dietetic Association.